Other titles in this series

THE BEST IN TENT CAMPING

A GUIDE FOR CAR CAMPERS WHO HATE RVs,
CONCRETE SLABS, AND LOUD PORTABLE STEREOS

ARIZONA

KIRSTIN OLMON AND KELLY PHILLIPS

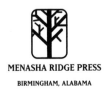

MENASHA RIDGE PRESS

BIRMINGHAM, ALABAMA

To all of the Forest Service and park rangers and volunteers who actually make our public lands work, and who must be doing it for love (it can't be the money). Thanks for sharing your stories with us.

Copyright © 2008 by Kirstin Olmon and Kelly Phillips
All rights reserved
Printed in the United States of America
Published by Menasha Ridge Press
Distributed by Publishers Group West
First edition, first printing

Library of Congress Cataloging-in-Publication Data

Olmon, Kirstin.
    The best in tent camping: Arizona: a guide for car campers who hate RVs, concrete slabs, and loud portable stereos/by Kirstin Olmon and Kelly Phillips. —1st ed.
    p. cm.
    Includes bibliographical references and index.
    ISBN-13: 978-0-89732-648-3 (alk. paper)
    ISBN-10: 0-89732-648-2 (alk. paper)
    1. Camping—Arizona—Guidebooks. 2. Camp sites, facilities, etc.—Arizona—Guidebooks.
3. Arizona—Guidebooks. I. Phillips, Kelly. II. Title.
    GV191.42.A7046 2008
    917.91'068—dc22

                              2008033040

Cover and text design by Ian Szymkowiak, Palace Press International, Inc.
Cover photo by Charles Liu
Cartography by Jennie Zehmer, Steve Jones, and Kelly Phillips
Indexing by Cynthia J. Coan

Menasha Ridge Press
P.O. Box 43673
Birmingham, Alabama 35243
www.menasharidge.com

TABLE OF CONTENTS

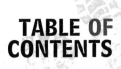

NORTHERN ARIZONA

CENTRAL ARIZONA

MOGOLLON RIM

TOP FIVE
ARIZONA
CAMPGROUNDS

BEST FOR BEAUTY
1 TUWEEP/TOROWEAP CAMPGROUND
2 NORTH RIM CAMPGROUND
26 FR 9350 DISPERSED AREA
36 KP CIENEGA CAMPGROUND
9 LOCKETT MEADOW CAMPGROUND

BEST FOR PRIVACY
35 BLUE CROSSING CAMPGROUND
37 HONEYMOON CAMPGROUND
34 PACHETA LAKE CAMPGROUND
23 UPPER PINAL CAMPGROUND
5 WINDY POINT RECREATION SITE

BEST FOR SPACIOUSNESS
26 FR 9350 DISPERSED AREA
37 HONEYMOON CAMPGROUND
8 FREIDLEIN PRAIRIE DISPERSED SITES
25 KNOLL LAKE CAMPGROUND
29 WORKMAN CREEK FALLS CAMPGROUND

BEST FOR QUIET
1 TUWEEP/TOROWEAP CAMPGROUND
45 ALAMO CANYON CAMPGROUND
5 WINDY POINT RECREATION SITE
4 CANYON VIEW CAMPGROUND
41 RIVERVIEW CAMPGROUND

BEST FOR SECURITY
27 FOOL HOLLOW LAKE RECREATION AREA
30 LYMAN LAKE STATE PARK
21 CHOLLA RECREATION SITE
4 CANYON VIEW CAMPGROUND
39 PICACHO PEAK STATE PARK

BEST FOR CLEANLINESS
16 BEAVER CREEK CAMPGROUND
27 FOOL HOLLOW LAKE RECREATION AREA
13 YAVAPAI CAMPGROUND
4 CANYON VIEW CAMPGROUND
3 DESERT VIEW CAMPGROUND

BEST FOR WHEELCHAIRS
27 FOOL HOLLOW LAKE RECREATION AREA
18 DESERT TORTOISE CAMPGROUND
39 PICACHO PEAK STATE PARK
13 YAVAPAI CAMPGROUND
7 DOGTOWN LAKE CAMPGROUND

BEST FOR FISHING
18 DESERT TORTOISE CAMPGROUND
32 CUTTHROAT CAMPGROUND
20 BURNT CORRAL RECREATION SITE
33 EAST FORK RECREATION AREA
16 BEAVER CREEK CAMPGROUND

BEST FOR HIKING
9 LOCKETT MEADOW CAMPGROUND
22 LOST DUTCHMAN STATE PARK
31 LOS BURROS CAMPGROUND
46 BOG SPRINGS CAMPGROUND
2 NORTH RIM CAMPGROUND

BEST FOR PADDLING
41 RIVERVIEW CAMPGROUND
30 LYMAN LAKE STATE PARK
18 DESERT TORTOISE CAMPGROUND
19 THE POINT CAMPGROUND
20 BURNT CORRAL RECREATION SITE

BEST FOR SWIMMING
10 MANZANITA CAMPGROUND
27 FOOL HOLLOW LAKE RECREATION AREA
20 BURNT CORRAL RECREATION SITE
30 LYMAN LAKE STATE PARK
18 DESERT TORTOISE CAMPGROUND

ABOUT THE AUTHORS

KIRSTIN OLMON AND KELLY PHILLIPS, transplants from other parts of the United States, both fell in love with Arizona from the first saguaro. Now they combine 19 years of experience roaming the Grand Canyon State's many landscapes. They live in Tempe, with a small menagerie, in a house that never gets cleaned on weekends, when trip planning often consists of just packing the dog into the pickup and picking a promising dotted line on the map. They never tire of providing vicarious adventures for friends and are thrilled to share Arizona's wonders with a wider audience in their first book.

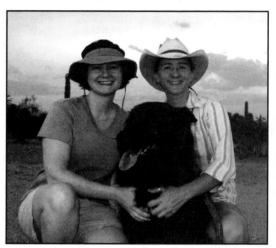

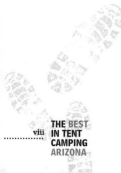

ACKNOWLEDGMENTS

- President Theodore Roosevelt and the other great conservationists of generations gone by, for making the effort to protect and preserve the land for future generations to enjoy
- The Civilian Conservation Corps for creating many of the wonderful campgrounds included in this book
- The folks at Menasha Ridge for giving us such a great opportunity
- Charles Liu for passing on to us the best possible excuse to go camping every weekend
- All of the folks in Take a Hike: Arizona hiking club, who shared their opinions and are buying this book (right, guys?)
- Our parents who, however unwittingly, raised us to wanderlust
- Our co-workers and friends who provided support and enthusiasm
- Laptops, wireless, and Google Docs, for making writing in camp, on the road, and in bed possible and practical
- The great state of Arizona, for providing countless hours of entertainment, sharing numerous secrets, and showing us beauty in many different forms

PREFACE

AS OUR PLANE MADE ITS BUMPY ARRIVAL at Sky Harbor International Airport, the kid next to us frowned out across the runway and mumbled resentfully, "I hate Arizona. It's so brown." We exchanged wry smiles, hearing the echo of so many other voices, even some long-term Phoenicians we know. Later we mulled over the injustice of it. Obviously this boy has never camped by the rushing Black River or seen the broad meadows and towering pines above the North Rim of the Grand Canyon. We planned exactly where we'd take this poor, misguided youth to show him just how green this state can be—up to the verdant crowns of the southern sky islands, the Chiricahuas, Pinaleños, Santa Ritas, Santa Catalinas, Huachucas; along the emerald riparian corridors of the Verde, Gila, and San Pedro rivers; and into the cool forests of the Mogollon Rim and the White Mountains.

Then we'd bring that kid to the desert again, to reveal to him the kaleidoscope of hues that it takes to make "brown" from an airplane window. In the spring, we'd hike him around the Superstitions and down to Picacho Peak to show him hillsides carpeted in yellow as the Mexican gold poppies and brittlebush bloom, and dotted with purple lupines and orange and pink mallows. He'd see the startling fuchsia, crimson, and lemon yellow of cholla, hedgehog, and prickly pear flowers against deep-green cactus skins. Finally, we'd make a grand tour of Sedona, Sycamore Canyon, the Painted Desert, and the Grand Canyon, to see all the vivid colors of the earth itself.

We have no idea who that boy was or how he ended up spending his time in Arizona, but this book is for him and all the kids out there like him.

Perhaps you're a visitor from elsewhere, or maybe you're a new Arizona resident wondering what you've gotten yourself into. If metro Phoenix is your main frame of reference, you might be forgiven for having some misgivings. There's an old joke that Arizona has only two seasons, hot and hotter, but cheer up—you can find spring, summer, winter, or fall within a five-hour drive at almost any time of the year. Somewhere in Arizona, there's a landscape and a climate to please almost everybody. What we've tried to do in this guide is help you find those places that will suit you best. We're making a few assumptions along the way: that you love the outdoors, that you favor peace and quiet but are sometimes willing to compromise, and that you appreciate a wide variety of different experiences. In short, that you're a lot like us.

Like so many Arizonans, we're imports from other climes, Kirstin from the lakes and snows of Minnesota and Kelly from the lush hills of Maryland. Kirstin knew from day one that she belonged here, while Kelly took some time to grow into a full appreciation of the desert. Family camping played a part of both our young lives, in tents, pop-ups, and cabins.

PREFACE

The leap to camping as adults came for both of us when we moved to the Grand Canyon State, where unparalleled natural diversity calls out to be explored.

Studies have shown that being in nature is good for your body and soul. This just makes sense in our modern world of superhighways, strip malls, and push-button electronic distractions. Congratulations on making the effort to tear yourselves (and especially your kids) away from the comfy chairs and glowing screens! The natural preserves and parks and wildlands need you as much as you need them. This is an era of budget squeezing and struggling to make ends meet for the Forest Service, the National Parks system, and state and county parks. Those of us who cherish these resources need to use and support them, to raise awareness of their value, and to raise another generation of responsible, educated, and enthusiastic campers—kids who get excited when they look out the airplane window.

INTRODUCTION

CHOOSING THE TOP 50

WHEN WE THINK OF THE BEST TENT CAMPING IN ARIZONA, the waterfalls of Havasu Canyon spring to mind, but the 11-mile hike, mule ride, or helicopter access meant it didn't make the cut. Since this book is written with car-campers in mind, we chose to only consider campgrounds that you could drive to (with the exception of one boat-access-only campground). Another book entirely could be written about the best backpacking camps in Arizona, but we haven't included any of those here. We included only official public campgrounds and tried to reach an equal balance of undeveloped and developed campgrounds. One of us must have her shower every day and the other would be perfectly happy to squat in the woods for weeks, so we think we represent both ends of the spectrum.

When we told other campers we were writing this book, smiles would cross their faces as they thought about their personal favorite places to pitch a tent. More often than not, if they chose to share their secret with us (knowing that we might reveal it to the public), they knew of a great location on public land with no more amenities than a fire ring and a great view. A startlingly high proportion of Arizona is public land, belonging to the Forest Service, the Bureau of Land Management, or the State of Arizona, and most of this is open to dispersed camping. Choose your own spot off the road or trail, maybe where someone else has camped or maybe not, with no fee, no facilities, no trash—strictly pack in/pack out. The wilderness is at your doorstep, and you may be all alone. We've kept our focus on official campgrounds and designated dispersed sites, and we leave it to you to discover Arizona's backcountry on your own. We've been told by Forest Service rangers that a lot of campers just want to know where they can camp for free and are uninterested in the amenities or the ambience. This isn't our target audience, but we have included many campgrounds that are free and indicate nearby dispersed camping locations.

We narrowed our choices among Arizona's many great campgrounds based on a number of factors. We divided the state into regions and looked for campgrounds that made an effort to give tenters something special, whether it be walk-in sites that have a better view of the lake, tent-only sections separated from the RVs, or other possibilities such as tenting on the beach or in the backcountry. In some regions we found too many good choices, but we tried to select the one or two that would be best for tenters. We looked for smaller campgrounds; the smaller the campground, the less likely a 30-foot fifth wheel will be your neighbor. Of course, the pioneer spirit is still alive and well in the West, and that means that you may find the modern equivalent of a Conestoga wagon almost anywhere, complete with a satellite dish and a patch of Astroturf by the door.

There are some areas of the state that we really wanted to include, such as Lake Mead, Lake Powell, Lake Havasu, Canyon de Chelley, Monument Valley, and the Colorado

Corridor. These are still terrific areas with their own special attractions, but the campgrounds we found either violated every stricture in our subtitle or didn't have designated camping that fit our standards. Tenters looking for solitude in these areas might want to rent a boat and camp on the shoreline or find a dispersed spot in the surrounding wilderness.

Some of the campgrounds we visited really defied our expectations. The managing agencies work hard to keep their Web sites and print information accurate and updated, but we found closed campgrounds, flooded campgrounds, and campgrounds that were unexpected gems. We hope that we've taken the legwork out of researching for you, and that our descriptions are clear enough for you to choose the campgrounds you'll like best. It's always a good idea to give the park or ranger district a call before you go for current conditions and unexpected events.

THE OVERVIEW MAP AND OVERVIEW-MAP KEY

Use the overview map on the inside front cover to assess the exact location of each campground. The campground's number appears not only on the overview map but also on the map key facing the overview map, in the table of contents, and on the profile's first page.

The book is organized by region, as indicated in the table of contents. A map legend that details the symbols found on the campground layout maps appears on the inside back cover.

CAMPGROUND-LAYOUT MAPS

Each profile contains a detailed campground-layout map that provides an overhead look at campground sites, internal roads, facilities, and other key items. Each campground entrance's GPS coordinates are included with each profile.

GPS CAMPGROUND-ENTRANCE COORDINATES

Readers can easily access all campgrounds in this book by using the directions given and the overview map, which shows at least one major road leading into the area. But for those who enjoy using the latest GPS technology to navigate, the necessary data has been provided. This book includes the GPS coordinates for each campground. To collect accurate map data, each campground was recorded with a handheld GPS unit. Data collected was then downloaded and plotted onto a digital USGS topo map. More accurately known as Universal Transverse Mercator (UTM) coordinates, the numbers index a specific point using a grid method. The survey datum used to arrive at the coordinates is WGS84. For readers who own a GPS unit, whether handheld or onboard a vehicle, the UTM coordinates provided with each campground description may be entered into the GPS unit. Just make sure your GPS unit is set to navigate using the UTM system in conjunction with WGS84 datum.

UTM COORDINATES: ZONE, EASTING, AND NORTHING

Within the UTM coordinates box within each campground description, there are three numbers labeled zone, easting, and northing. Here is an example from Desert View Campground at Grand Canyon National Park.

UTM Zone (WGS84) 12S
Easting 425556
Northing 3988810

The zone number (12) refers to one of the 60 longitudinal zones (vertical) of a map using the UTM projection. Each zone is 6° wide. The zone letter (S) refers to one of the 20 latitudinal zones (horizontal) that span from 80° South to 84° North.

The easting number (425556) references in meters how far east the point is from the zero value for eastings, which runs north-south through Greenwich, England. Increasing easting coordinates on a topo map or on your GPS screen indicate you are moving east; decreasing easting coordinates indicate you are moving west. Since lines of longitude converge at the poles, they are not parallel as lines of latitude are. This means that the distance between Full Easting Coordinates is 1,000 meters near the equator but becomes smaller as you travel farther north or south; the difference is small enough to be ignored, but only until you reach the polar regions.

In the Northern Hemisphere, the northing number (3988810) references in meters how far you are from the equator. Above the equator, northing coordinates increase by 1,000 meters between each parallel line of latitude (east-west lines). On a topo map or GPS receiver, increasing northing numbers indicate you are traveling north.

In the Southern Hemisphere, the northing number references how far you are from a latitude line that is 10 million meters south of the equator. Below the equator, northing coordinates decrease by 1,000 meters between each line of latitude. On a topo map, decreasing northing coordinates indicate you are traveling south.

THE RATING SYSTEM

The campgrounds were pitted against each other, not against other campgrounds in the state. So if two campgrounds have similar rankings, you can expect similar experiences. We were tough graders and gave out few fives, but we feel that each campground we've included is superlative in its own way.

BEAUTY

Beauty, of course, is in the eye of the beholder, but we gave higher marks for panoramic views or proximity to a lake or river. A campground that blended in well with the environment scored well, as did areas with remarkable wildlife or geology. Well-grown vegetation and nicely laid-out sites also upped the ratings.

PRIVACY

For privacy we looked at the number of sites, the amount of screening between them, and physical distance from one another. Other factors include the presence of nearby trails or day-use areas, and proximity to a town or city that would provide regular day-use traffic.

SPACIOUSNESS

Spaciousness is both a matter of actual space and of the feeling of having elbow room. We checked the separation of tent spots, picnic tables, cooking areas, and vehicles. We adjusted our marks based on whether activity areas and tent pads were defined or bordered, and scored higher for the potential to spread out. We also gave campgrounds with plenty of space between the sites a higher rating.

QUIET

The quietness of the campground will of course depend on who your neighbors are and when you are visiting. We took into consideration our experience at the site, the nearness of roads, the proximity of towns and cities, the probable number of RVs, the likelihood of noisy ATVs or boats, and whether a campground host is available or willing to enforce the quiet hours. If we heard a campground had a reputation for rowdiness or if we witnessed a ruckus ourselves, we removed it from consideration.

SECURITY

How you determine a campground's security will depend on who you view as the greater risk: other people or the wilderness. The more remote the campground, the less likely you are to run into opportunistic crime, but the more remote the campground, the harder it is to get help in case of an accident or confrontation. We tried to reach a balance by considering whether there was a campground host or resident park ranger, how close your neighbors were to your site, how much day traffic the campground received, how close the campground was to a town or city, and whether there was cell-phone coverage or some type of pay phone or emergency call button.

CLEANLINESS

A campground's appearance often depends on who was there right before you and how your visit coincides with the maintenance schedule. In general, we gave higher marks to those campgrounds with hosts who cleaned up regularly. We also gave high marks in the rare case of odor-free toilets. At unhosted campgrounds, we looked for trash receptacles and evidence that sites were cleared and that signs and buildings were kept repaired. We didn't necessarily mark down for a single visitor's garbage left at a site, but we definitely did for the old trash in shrubbery and along trails that indicates infrequent cleaning.

FIRST-AID KIT

A useful first-aid kit may contain more items than you might think necessary. These are just the basics. Prepackaged kits in waterproof bags (Atwater Carey and Adventure Medical make them) are available. As a preventive measure, take along sunscreen and insect repellent. Even though quite a few items are listed here, they pack down into a small space:

Ace bandages or Spenco joint wraps

Adhesive bandages, such as Band-Aids

Antibiotic ointment (*Neosporin or the generic equivalent*)

Antiseptic or disinfectant, such as Betadine or hydrogen peroxide

Aspirin or acetaminophen

Benadryl or the generic equivalent, diphenhydramine (*in case of allergic reactions*)

Butterfly-closure bandages

Comb and tweezers (*for removing stray cactus needles from your skin*)

Emergency poncho

Epinephrine in a prefilled syringe (*for people known to have severe allergic reactions to such things as bee stings*)

Gauze (one roll)

Gauze compress pads (*six 4- x 4-inch pads*)

LED flashlight or headlamp

Matches or pocket lighter

Mirror for signaling passing aircraft

Moleskin/Spenco "Second Skin"

Pocketknife or multipurpose tool

Waterproof first-aid tape

Whistle (*it's more effective in signaling rescuers than your voice*)

ROADS AND VEHICLES

While doing the research for this book and bumping along dirt roads all over the state, we reset our standards for what constitutes a good road. We consider a good road to be well-graded dirt, wide, with few rocks or dips, where we can clip along at 30 mph. We traveled to all of these campgrounds in a stock 4WD Toyota T100 and after driving more than 12,000 miles, we've only had to replace the shocks and brakes, tighten a few loose bolts, and fix one flat tire.

High clearance gives you the ability to cruise most of the state's back roads and a 4WD can get you out of a sticky situation, but the majority of these campgrounds can be reached by a careful driver in a standard sedan when the roads are dry. Road conditions can change quickly with the weather, so be sure to call 511 or the phone number in the campground entry to get a report on road conditions. Obey all traffic signs, and keep in mind that vehicles driving uphill have the right-of-way on narrow roads.

Arizona's hundreds of miles of forest roads can open up a lot of backcountry for those of us who aren't long-distance backpackers. Get a good, detailed map, like the DeLorme Gazetteer, if you intend to travel the back roads, make sure your vehicle's in good shape, and carry an emergency kit with plenty of water.

CAMPGROUND COURTESY

We were asked by more than one campground host to include a comment about camp-ground courtesy in our book. This stuff is common sense, but like a lot of common sense, it bears repeating. Be aware of the quiet hours, especially when pulling into a campground after dark. Avoid shining your headlights or flashlights into other campsites as you are searching for a spot. And please turn down your car stereo; that bass beat carries very well in the night. Always walk on the designated paths and roads, and respect the privacy of your neigh-bors by not strolling through their site to get to the restrooms. You'll also reduce damage to the foliage and keep the campground green by sticking to the main trail. Please clean up after yourself. In Girl Scouts, we were taught to scavenge around the campsite picking up every piece of trash we could find, even if it wasn't ours. Make cleaning up into a game with your kids: whoever packs out the most twist-ties, pop tops, and gum wrappers is the winner.

CAMPING IN ARIZONA

Many people fear rattlesnakes and scorpions but practically flirt with Arizona's real danger—the sun. It gets hot here, and don't let anyone tell you that because it's a dry heat it doesn't count. Dehydration and heat exhaustion commonly afflict the unprepared, unwary, or merely overconfident. Be sure to carry three liters of water per person per day and drink it. Consider investing in a Camelbak or Platypus water container since having water more accessible increases the likelihood that you will actually drink it. One trick we discovered was to fill empty two-liter soda bottles or plastic juice bottles with water and freeze them. Use them in your cooler instead of ice cubes. When the ice melts, you have an emergency supply of water for drinking, or you can use it to put out your campfire. Wear a wide-brimmed hat, sunscreen, and sunglasses. Wear lightweight, long-sleeved shirts and pants if you expect to be in the sun all day. It seems counterintuitive, but you will stay cooler if you protect your skin from the sun by wearing more clothing.

Be prepared for cool nights as well. Once the sun sets out in the desert, it can get cold fast. Bring layers and expect the unexpected from Arizona's weather. We've included campgrounds from 1,700 to 9,000 feet in elevation. You'll experience major changes in temperature, weather, and plant life as you change elevation. Knowing the elevation of a region will give you an idea of what conditions to prepare for.

The summer monsoon season happens from mid-July through early September. Expect heavy afternoon rains nearly every day, which can sometimes turn to hail at higher elevations. Bring a tarp to cover your gear and carry a poncho or rain jacket. These pouring rains often fall on soil that's too dry or stony to absorb them, making monsoon season prime flash-flood time. Always place your tent with an eye to drainage and never take chances crossing a flooded wash, no matter how big your vehicle is.

The rainy season is also part of the fire season, since lightning strikes spark many forest fires. Many others, sadly, are caused by careless people. Don't make yourself famous—always douse your campfires completely. We carry a 6-gallon jug of water in our truck specifically for that purpose. Keep your campfire under control and below knee level, or better yet, use a gas stove, which does less damage to the ground and roots beneath. Seasonal fire restrictions are no joke, and the penalties for disregarding them are serious.

You may be concerned about encountering Arizona's more infamous wildlife, such as rattlesnakes, scorpions, black bears, wolves, coyotes, and mountain lions. Your chances of even glimpsing most of these critters are actually pretty slim—they'll usually go out of their way to avoid you.

Follow these few simple rules to reduce the chance of an up-close-and-personal experience:

- Clean up after yourself in camp. Put all food and toiletries in your vehicle or a bear-proof container or hang them from a tree, but don't keep them in your tent!
- Don't leave your shoes or other gear outside of your tent overnight or be sure to shake them out before using them.
- Keep track of your kids and leash your pets.
- Don't stick your hands and feet into dark crevices.

If you should encounter a wild animal, give it plenty of space and don't provoke it. You are much more likely to be endangered by elk and deer (and cows!) while you're on the road. As the four-part warning signs along some of Arizona's highways say: "Elk are large, In herds they run, Across the highway, Don't hit one!"

Be sure to tell someone of your travel plans and keep in touch. We're in the habit of sending Kirstin's sister a text message once we decide where we we're going to camp, then checking in when we arrive home safely. This can be lifesaving if something untoward happens, and it also keeps your loved ones from worrying.

PERMITS AND ACCESS

If you like to explore Arizona as we do, you might benefit by purchasing an America the Beautiful National Parks and Federal Recreational Lands Annual Pass (for obvious reasons, everybody refers to it as just the Interagency Pass). This replaces the Golden Eagle pass and is available through the National Park Service. The current cost is $80 per year, but it covers entrance to all national parks (including the Grand Canyon's $25 entrance fee) and national monuments, and most fee areas on land managed by the Forest Service, the Bureau of Land Management, and the U.S. Fish and Wildlife Service. Many fee areas in Sedona will also accept this pass in place of the local Red Rock pass. The pass does not cover camping fees but we've found it to be very cost-effective on entrance fees alone.

The Tonto National Forest, which has a lot of heavily used recreation areas near Phoenix, has a slightly different pass program. The Tonto Pass is required at many recreation sites, especially in ranger districts close to Phoenix. Check with the Forest Service prior to heading out, since daily hangtags can be purchased from Forest Service offices, online, or from many local retail stores, but *not* at the recreation sites. Each pass has scratch-off date blocks so you can buy them in advance and mark them on the day of use. The daily pass is $6 per vehicle and $4 per watercraft. You can purchase an annual Tonto Upgrade Decal for $15 if you already own an Interagency Pass. This covers your daily fee, but not your camping fee, so you'll still need a daily hangtag if you want to camp.

The Arizona state parks annual pass is $50 and covers your entrance fee to all of the state recreational and historical parks in Arizona, with the exception of the three parks around Lake Havasu City on weekends. This pass does not cover your camping fees, and your entrance fee is waived when you camp, so purchase this pass if you plan to visit, but not camp, at several parks through the year.

The National Interagency and Arizona State Parks passes between them will give you access to most of the public lands and parks in Arizona, which is why Kirstin always asks for them for Christmas. Consider giving your family the gift of travel while supporting the parks. Many regional and county parks throughout the state also issue annual passes, but they're park-specific. You may also want to purchase the $15 State Land Recreational Permit that allows you to hike, camp, or drive off-road on state trust land. It's available from the Arizona State Land Department. You won't need one to camp at any of the campgrounds we've included in the book, but it wouldn't hurt to carry a permit if you plan to drive off-road often. Visit **www.land.state.az.us** to download a permit application.

Most of Arizona's Native American reservations are self-governing territories with their own rules and regulations for outdoor activities and backcountry travel. If you would like to spend time on Native American lands, check in with the local tribal authorities for specific information.

Now that your windshield is decked out in passes and your head is full of facts, take this handy book and get out there. The best tent camping in Arizona is waiting for you!

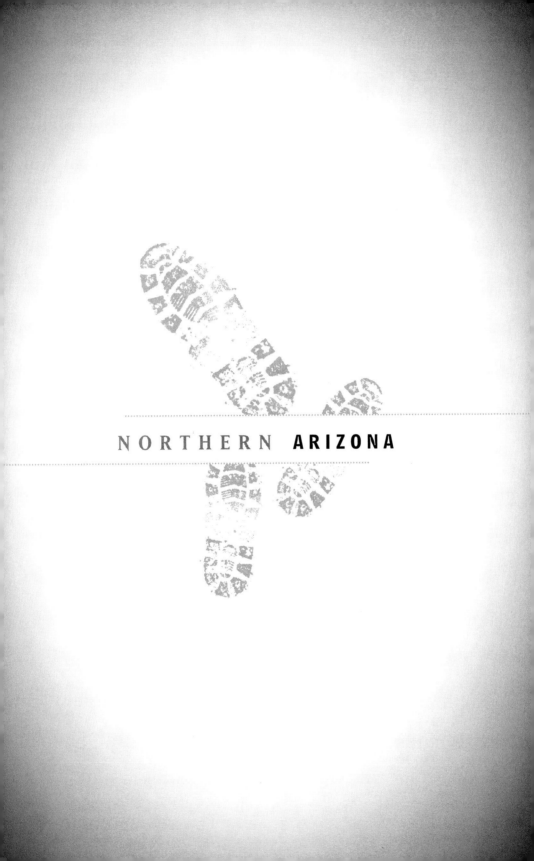

NORTHERN ARIZONA

1
TUWEEP/TOROWEAP CAMPGROUND

AS YOU LEAVE THE HIGHWAY, signs read "prim-itive road, use at your own risk." Other signs warn that no services are available; the Park Service recommends you bring extra water, food, gas-oline, spare tires, and tools. The beginning of the drive is sandy, and flocks of sparrows flitter away to avoid your trailing dust plume. As the long washboard road winds on it may be rutted or peppered with rocks and tire-thumping potholes. Take your time (allow two to three hours) and enjoy the scenery as it subtly changes from scrub brush to grassy plains to juniper-covered hillsides.

This is nothing like entering Grand Canyon National Park at the South or North Rim. There's no entrance station, and (you may be pleasantly surprised to learn) no $25 fee. You can stop at the tiny Tuweep Ranger Station to pick up hiking information or an area brochure, but if you require backcountry permits, it's best to get them in advance. The ranger who lives here year-round also has patrol duties and may not be avail-able. The campground is only 5.4 miles past the station, but it's the most difficult stretch of the road. Here the slickrock is exposed, and large, sometimes sharp, rocks are waiting to eat your tires. Once you turn left into the campground, hop out of your vehicle, celebrate your achievement, and check for loose bolts!

The campground rests on deep shelves carved out of the sandstone of the Toroweap formation by aeons of erosion. All of the sites have tremendous views looking out over the pinyon-studded slickrock toward the varie-gated walls of the canyon. The sites are numbered and well spaced, each with a picnic table and fire pit. Gather-ing wood is prohibited, so bring your own, especially if you are coming in fall or winter. Camping is free and no reservations are required, so take your pick of the sites, but if you're dependent on stakes to support your tent, scout carefully—the loose soil is thin over the stone.

> *From here, you can look straight down 3,000 feet into the steepest, narrowest part of the Grand Canyon and see the Colorado River below.*

RATINGS

Beauty: ✿ ✿ ✿ ✿ ✿
Privacy: ✿ ✿ ✿ ✿
Spaciousness: ✿ ✿ ✿ ✿ ✿
Quiet: ✿ ✿ ✿ ✿ ✿
Security: ✿ ✿ ✿ ✿
Cleanliness: ✿ ✿ ✿ ✿

The first three sites are to the right of the entrance, on slightly higher and more open ground. Site 1 is large, but the uneven and rocky ground might make for an uncomfortable night unless you have a good mattress. Try for site 2, where you have a terrific view and are likely to get some afternoon shade from the pinyon pines.

Turn left to reach sites 4 through 10, where the curve of the rim forms a sheltered basin. The camp road traces the edge of the bare, stone shelf, so pick your route carefully and watch for grooves in the rock where others have scraped. Climb two or three stone steps to get up to sites 4 and 5, where a rock wall and pinyon pines provide afternoon shade, the tent pads are cleared, and the world spreads out in front of you. Adding a gently civilized touch, someone has done a little Xeriscaping, and white stones ring nearby agaves and yuccas. Site 6 is tucked in the bend of the rock rim, with surrounding walls and a 90-degree view across the valley. Underneath the large, rock awning at site 7 you can set up your tent behind the trees and brush and easily imagine life as a cliff dweller. This site might also be a good choice during the July to September thunderstorm season. Continue around the rim, and site 8 sits underneath a huge mushrooming boulder with lots of afternoon shade. Nearby, site 9 is also tucked underneath projecting rock. There's a touch of history in this sheltered spot—stacked rocks in natural openings in the boulders create walls with windows, and peeling plaster and an old stove pipe attest to the effort of a bygone cowboy, prospector, or hermit. Out in front of site 9, two picnic tables and a fire ring constitute the group site 10. There are no cleared pads, but you'll have plenty of room on the flat rock to pitch several tents.

Once you have chosen your site, hike or drive the mile to the spectacular Toroweap Overlook. From here, you can look straight down 3,000 feet into the steepest, narrowest part of the Grand Canyon and see the Colorado River below. Even from this height you can hear

KEY INFORMATION

ADDRESS:	Grand Canyon National Park, P.O. Box 129 Grand Canyon, AZ 86023
OPERATED BY:	National Park Service
INFORMATION:	(928) 638-7888, www.nps.gov/grca
OPEN:	Year-round if accessible
SITES:	10
EACH SITE:	Picnic table, fire ring
ASSIGNMENT:	First come, first served; reservations accepted for group site
REGISTRATION:	None required
FACILITIES:	Composting toilets, group site, resident park ranger, and emergency phone located at Tuweep Ranger Station
PARKING:	At campsites
FEE:	Free
ELEVATION:	4,600 feet
RESTRICTIONS:	*Pets:* On leash only, not permitted on Lava Falls Trail, Tuckup Trail, or anywhere in inner canyon. *Fires:* In fire rings only. *Alcohol:* Permitted. *Vehicles:* RVs and trailers not recommended; high clearance recommended; 2 vehicles per site; ATVs prohibited; off-road travel prohibited. *Other:* Pack in/pack out; firearms prohibited; firewood-gathering prohibited; 8 people per site; collecting, destroying, or disturbing any natural resource prohibited; no drinking water available; quiet hours 10 p.m.–6 a.m.

MAP

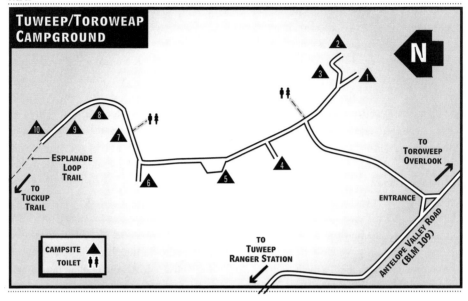

TUWEEP/TOROWEAP CAMPGROUND

ESPLANADE LOOP TRAIL

TO TUCKUP TRAIL

TO TOROWEEP OVERLOOK

ENTRANCE

TO TUWEEP RANGER STATION

ANTELOPE VALLEY ROAD (BLM 109)

CAMPSITE
TOILET

N

the roar of Lava Falls, the most dangerous rapid on the river. Be sure to watch your step and keep a close eye on children; there are no barriers here. Old maps show two more campsites at the overlook, but these have since been converted to a day-use-only picnic area. You can hike all the way down to the Colorado River from here—switchbacking 2,500 feet in 1.5 miles—following the shortest trail from rim to river in the entire park. This is not a simple day hike, though. The unmaintained trail is difficult to follow, the rock underfoot is unstable, and the climb is brutal in warmer weather. If you're interested in hiking the Lava Falls Trail, get the information you'll need to do it safely from the Park Service. For a less-treacherous hike, take the Tuckup Trail and see if you can find the ancient pictographs, some 6 feet tall, called Gordon's Panel or the Shamans' Gallery. If the campground is full, backtrack outside the park boundary for dispersed camping. You'll discover some particularly nice spots among the junipers along the Mount Trumbull Road. The road continues west and climbs into a ponderosa forest near the 6,500-foot peak of Mount Trumbull, an extinct volcano. In this rarely visited area, the 5-mile hike to the peak abounds with wildlife. This scenic drive eventually winds up in St. George, Utah.

GETTING THERE

From Fredonia, take AZ 389 west 7 miles to Antelope Valley Road (BLM Road 109). Turn left and continue south 61 miles to campground.

GPS COORDINATES

Zone 12S

Easting 314714

Northing 4010629

North 36° 13' 22.02"

West 113° 3' 41.40"

2
NORTH RIM CAMPGROUND

> *Camp at one of several scenic points and have the entire area to yourself.*

ARIZONA ABOUNDS WITH great spots to pitch a tent, but for solitude and sheer, stunning beauty, nothing beats the north rim of the Grand Canyon. The North Rim is the less-known, less-popular, harder-to-reach, but just-as-spectacular way to view America's most famous natural wonder. Of the 5 million people who visit the Grand Canyon every year, 90 percent go to the South Rim and see the canyon from the overlooks. The North Rim sees far fewer visitors, with places to camp where you might even have the grandeur of the grandest canyon all to yourself.

There's one developed campground inside the park, with 83 tent and RV sites located right on the rim, plus a lodge with cabins for rent. Both the lodge and campground fill up during summer, especially on weekends, so reservations are highly recommended. Only a few premium sites have a view of the canyon, so when booking, try to get sites 10, 11, 14 through 16, 18, or group site 2. Transept Trail, the 1.5-mile hike along the rim to North Rim Lodge, begins between sites 15 and 16. If the premium sites are not available, try to reserve one of the more-private sites along the outer loop on the eastern side. The sites are underneath ponderosa pines with little screening undergrowth. Don't bother with the tent-only loop—it's a parking lot. Near North Rim Campground you'll find several amenities that are blessings to weary hikers, including hot showers, laundry facilities, and a general store with simple groceries and souvenirs. Other services include a bookstore, interpretive programs, gas, and a dump station. After the park road has closed for the winter, you can hike, snowshoe, or ski in to use the campground on a first-come, first-served basis with a backcountry permit, but services are limited.

If you're looking for even less of a crowd, you have another option. Inside the national park boundary,

RATINGS

Beauty: ✿ ✿ ✿ ✿ ✿
Privacy: ✿ ✿ ✿ ✿
Spaciousness: ✿ ✿ ✿
Quiet: ✿ ✿ ✿ ✿ ✿
Security: ✿ ✿ ✿ ✿
Cleanliness: ✿ ✿ ✿ ✿ ✿

you must camp at designated campsites only. What most people don't realize is that you can camp at several scenic points with a backcountry permit and have the entire area to yourself, since the park limits the number of permits issued. If you're up for a rough 17-mile drive, Point Sublime offers three sites with eastern views of Confucius Temple, Mencius Temple, Osiris Temple, and Dragon Head—with a bonus of great sunrises. Point Sublime even boasts a composting toilet with open-air charm. Primitive at-large camping is available on the Walhalla Plateau, near the Widforss Trail, and in a few other areas, and there's a single designated spot right on the rim down the 2-mile trail to Cape Final. The earlier you plan, the more likely your first choice will be granted. The backcountry office can give you even more options; they answer the phone and make reservations 1 p.m. to 5 p.m. Monday through Friday. These lines are often busy; the best days to call are Thursday and Friday. If you're more of a last-minute type, drop by the permit office at the north rim to check for availabilities. Dog owners take note: you'll have to convince the rangers you're not taking your pets into the canyon, and they still may not be allowed in the backcountry.

There's also terrific dispersed camping in the Kaibab National Forest surrounding the park boundary. Lookout points such as Marbleview, Crazy Jug, and Dog Point require only a drive down a bumpy road to reach overlooks nearly as spectacular as any in the park. Dispersed camping in the national forest is free, and pets are allowed as long as you clean up after them. You must be self-contained since there are no toilets or trash service, but you also have no fees, permits, or reservations to worry about. You can build a campfire in the national forest (with adequate precautions), but not in the national park's backcountry.

KEY INFORMATION

ADDRESS: Grand Canyon National Park, P.O. Box 129, Grand Canyon, AZ 86023
OPERATED BY: National Park Service
INFORMATION: (928) 638-7888, www.nps.gov/grca
OPEN: Mid-May to mid-October
SITES: 87
EACH SITE: Picnic table, fire ring
ASSIGNMENT: First come, first served; reservations available by calling (877) 444-6777 or visiting www.recreation.gov
REGISTRATION: Check in at kiosk
FACILITIES: Vault toilets, flush toilets, dump station, hot showers, pay phones, laundry, day-use area, amphitheater, interpretive activities and programs, group area, drinking fountains, firewood, campground host, handicap-accessible sites and toilets, general store
PARKING: At campsites
FEE: $18–$25, plus $25 seven-day entrance fee
ELEVATION: 8,300 feet
RESTRICTIONS: *Pets:* On leash only; prohibited on trails, in wilderness areas, and below rim. Pets may not be left unattended, and there are no kennels on the North Rim. *Fires:* In fire rings only. *Alcohol:* Permitted. *Vehicles:* 2 vehicles per site; vehicle pulling a trailer counts as 2 vehicles. *Other:* Firewood gathering prohibited; 6-person limit per site; 3-tent limit per site; 7-day stay limit; quiet hours 10 p.m.–6.am.; checkout 10 a.m.

MAP

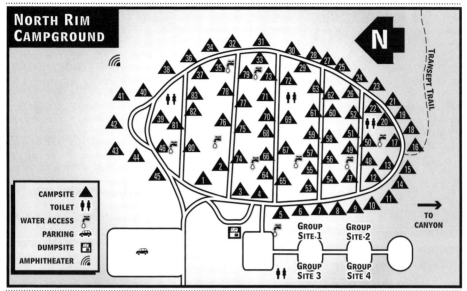

NORTH RIM CAMPGROUND

CAMPSITE ▲
TOILET 👫
WATER ACCESS 🚰
PARKING 🚗
DUMPSITE 🗑
AMPHITHEATER 📡

TO CANYON →

TRANSEPT TRAIL

GROUP SITE·1
GROUP SITE·2
GROUP SITE 3
GROUP SITE 4

GETTING THERE

From Jacob Lake, take AZ 67 south 30 miles to the park entrance. Continue south 12 miles to the turnoff to the campground. Turn right and head west to the campground entrance.

GPS COORDINATES

Zone 12S
Easting 404663
Northing 4007801
North 36° 12' 37.26"
West 112° 03' 38.16"

Several forested trails along the rim offer great views of the canyon, including the 10-mile Widforss Trail, the 5-mile Uncle Jim Trail, and the 4-mile Cape Final Trail. If you plan to hike into the Grand Canyon on the North Kaibab Trail, be sure to call the backcountry office and plan ahead. You must have a permit to hike overnight, and it is recommended that you not hike more than 10 miles in one day, nor between 10 a.m. and 4 p.m. in the summer. If you plan to hike all the way down the canyon to the Colorado River, you must spend the night at Cottonwood Camp, 7 miles below the rim. The Grand Canyon is an amazing place to visit, so make your visit a safe one. Know the dangers of the canyon—stay a safe distance from the edges, remain on the trails, and drink plenty of water and eat salty snacks while hiking.

One last note: seeing both sides of the canyon in one trip may be difficult—it's only 10 miles across as the crow flies, but it takes at least five hours to drive the 220 miles from the South Rim to the North Rim.

3
DESERT VIEW CAMPGROUND

The campground to go to if you are looking for a quieter experience at one of the world's largest tourist attractions.

NO BOOK ABOUT THE BEST CAMPING in Arizona would be complete without mentioning Grand Canyon National Park. One of the seven natural wonders of the world, it is Arizona's main claim to fame and receives 5 million visitors each year. That can mean a lot of chaos and congestion. Luckily, most of those people concentrate near Grand Canyon Village on the South Rim and don't explore the rest of the park. You can still have a peaceful experience at one of the world's largest tourist attractions.

The South Rim offers two developed campgrounds—Mather and Desert View. Mather's 320 campsites are near Grand Canyon Village, the South Rim's hub, with everything you could possibly need. It's open year-round, and reservations are strongly recommended from March 1 through mid-November. Desert View, open seasonally on a first-come first-served basis, is the campground to go to if you are looking for something quieter.

Approaching from the village along Desert View Drive, you pass some of the park's most famous viewpoints, while the flora changes from tall pines to open pinyon/juniper woodland. You won't see the canyon from the campground, but just a short distance away is Desert View overlook, site of the Watchtower. Climb to the top, the highest point on the South Rim, for incredible views. The tower itself is a historical landmark, a Pueblo-inspired creation of the Fred Harvey Company's remarkable architect, Mary Jane Elizabeth Colter. You'll also find a gas station, convenience store, snack bar, and gift shop here; close by are the Ranger Station and the east entrance to the park.

In the campground, 50 sites line one long, narrow, paved loop. The sites inside the loop back up to each other, so you don't have much privacy, but the sites on the outside of the loop are more spacious. The junipers and other low scrub provide some screening between

RATINGS

Beauty: ✩ ✩ ✩
Privacy: ✩ ✩ ✩
Spaciousness: ✩ ✩ ✩
Quiet: ✩ ✩ ✩
Security: ✩ ✩ ✩ ✩
Cleanliness: ✩ ✩ ✩ ✩ ✩

most sites, and all of them have a cleared tent area. We think the better sites, inside and out, are on the second half of the loop. Sites 22, 38, and 42 have particularly good screening and separation from their neighbors, and site 29 is spacious and shady, set well back from a generous pullout. The most private site in the campground, and the best choice for summer, is site 46. It's small, but has a complete screen of junipers and a deeply shaded tent spot.

Ravens keep a close eye on you in camp, and if you turn your back, the swoosh of big, black wings will signal the disappearance of anything that looks like food. Given enough time, a Grand Canyon raven will even unzip a backpack and rifle through it. For your sake and theirs, keep a tidy camp kitchen and store your food well.

Large RVs are encouraged to stay at Trailer Village, but smaller RVs, often rentals, are everywhere. The park has set longer quiet hours than you'll find in many camp-grounds: generator use is limited to 8 a.m. to 8 p.m., and loud music is prohibited at all times. Your fellow campers may come from all over the globe, so say hi and enjoy meeting someone new and different.

The best way to enjoy your visit to the Grand Canyon is to plan ahead. Peruse the NPS Web site and call the information centers. Study up, especially if you intend to enter the canyon itself. Below the rim, the canyon is a uniquely rewarding and uniquely dangerous place to hike. You descend while you're fresh and rested, and only when you're already tired do you face the reality of climbing back up. Throw in the dry, desert climate and the 20- to 40-degree difference between rim and Canyon temperatures, and you have a recipe for hun-dreds of rescues and several deaths every year.

With a little extra planning and effort, you might have a campsite with a view of the canyon all to yourself. You must have a permit to camp outside of designated campgrounds,

KEY INFORMATION

ADDRESS:	Grand Canyon National Park, P.O. Box 129, Grand Canyon, AZ 86023
OPERATED BY:	National Park Service
INFORMATION:	(928) 638-7888, www.nps.gov/grca
OPEN:	May 1–mid-October
SITES:	50
EACH SITE:	Picnic table, fire ring
ASSIGNMENT:	First come, first served; no reservations
REGISTRATION:	On-site self-registration
FACILITIES:	Flush toilets, water spigots, trash, recycling; gas, pay phone, general store nearby
PARKING:	At campsites
FEE:	$12 plus $25 7-day park entrance fee
ELEVATION:	7,500 feet
RESTRICTIONS:	*Pets:* On leash only; prohibited below rim, in park lodging, or on park buses. There is a kennel at South Rim, reservations recommended. Pets are not permitted on North Rim trails. *Fires:* In fire rings only. *Alcohol:* Permitted. *Vehicles:* 30-foot length limit; no ATVs; 2-vehicle or 1-RV/trailer limit. *Other:* 7-day stay limit; bear-country food-storage restrictions; fire-arms prohibited; 6 people per site; 2-tent limit; quiet hours 10 p.m.–8 a.m.; checkout 11 a.m.; no firewood gathering; mountain lion country

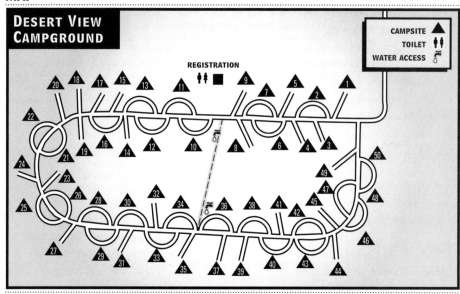

DESERT VIEW CAMPGROUND

CAMPSITE ▲
TOILET
WATER ACCESS

REGISTRATION

but backcountry camping can be found both above and below the rim. If you're up for a backpack experience, but don't want to challenge the canyon itself, try Cape Solitude. At-large camping is permitted almost anywhere along the 15.6-mile hike. To explore other possibilities, call the backcountry office between 1 p.m. and 5 p.m. Monday through Friday, and the rangers will help you plan your ideal trip. Dispersed camping is also available at no cost in the Kaibab National Forest south of the park border.

Don't ignore the most popular parts of the park—the Park Service has worked hard to make visiting an enjoyable experience, and the lodges and shops at the village have history and charms of their own to explore. A nice way to see the busiest part of the canyon is from the partially paved Rim Trail, which stretches from Hermit's Rest in the west to Yaki Point. You can park at one of the viewpoints, walk all or a portion of the trail, and catch the shuttle bus back to your car. The free, alternative-fuel shuttles don't come as far as Desert View, but if you've come to the canyon via the Grand Canyon Railway (for more details see profile 7, Dogtown Lake), there is taxi service from the village.

GETTING THERE

From Flagstaff to the east entrance station, take US 89 north 65 miles to AZ 64. Turn left and drive west 50 miles to the east entrance station. Turn right into the campground.

From Flagstaff to Grand Canyon Village, take US 180 west 51 miles to AZ 64. Turn right and drive north 31 miles to the South Rim entrance station.

GPS COORDINATES

Zone 12S
Easting 425556
Northing 3988810
North 36° 2' 27.54"
West 111° 49' 35.04"

4
CANYON VIEW CAMPGROUND

> *These are among the best-preserved cliff dwellings in the country.*

THE NAVAJO NATION IS BEST KNOWN for the austere beauty of the Painted Desert, with its rough, red mountains and color-striped mineral badlands, and the stark magnificence of Monument Valley. Between the two, a surprise awaits in the pinyon-brushed hills near Kayenta—the lovely gem of Navajo National Monument. Established in 1909 and managed by the National Park Service, it protects three Ancestral Puebloan ruins—Betatakin, Keet Seel, and Inscription House. Built in the 13th century by the Hisatsinom, ancient ancestors of today's Hopi clans, these are among the best-preserved cliff dwellings in the country, culturally important for the Hopi, Zuni, Paiute, and Diné (Navajo) peoples.

When you first enter the park, stop at the visitor center to chat with the rangers, many of whom are Diné, and see the interpretive displays and ancient pottery. Artisans frequently demonstrate traditional crafts such as rug weaving, and next door you'll find a gift shop specializing in silver Navajo jewelry. The visitor center also offers flush toilets, drinking fountains, a pay phone, and a picnic area. You can crawl into the nearby sweathouse and image what it was like to bathe without water and dry off with sand. Stand in the hogan, an example of traditional Navajo housing, then head out to pitch your own tent.

With two no-fee campgrounds at the monument, you can choose the amenities that best suit you. Sunset View Campground provides paved roads and parking tabs, handicap-accessible spots, flush toilets, a service sink and gray water disposal, and of course, views of the setting sun. We recommend Canyon View, designed for tent campers who prefer a simpler, more secluded experience. Take a right as you leave the visitor center parking lot, toward the Keet Seel Trail. As you leave the pavement behind you, look for the employee housing

RATINGS

Beauty: ✿ ✿ ✿ ✿
Privacy: ✿ ✿ ✿
Spaciousness: ✿ ✿ ✿
Quiet: ✿ ✿ ✿ ✿ ✿
Security: ✿ ✿ ✿ ✿
Cleanliness: ✿ ✿ ✿ ✿ ✿

on the left and the corral on the right. The Keet Seel trailhead parking is just below the entrance to the campground.

A slender thread of sites, Canyon View sits on a ridge between the canyon containing Keet Seel ruin and Shonto Plateau. Almost all of the sites command a canyon view. You'll find only patchy shade in the pinyon-juniper woodland, but at nearly 7,300 feet elevation, the mornings and evenings prove to be cool and comfortable. Most of the sites are well screened. The first site is very private and set apart with a generous pull-through. Site 2 has a shallower pulloff but offers good morning shade, as do all of the sites on the east side of the road. Sites 7 through 9, 12, and 13 provide the best view of the Betatakin Canyon. Sites 10 and 11 are group sites, available for free on a first-come, first-served basis. Situated in the center of the loop at the end of the line of campsites, site 11 is open and uncomfortably rocky. A large group here would affect sites 9, 12, and 13, which are otherwise quite nice. Site 10 is the better group site, being off to the side with a large, smooth area for tents.

While you won't have a campground host, signs with emergency numbers are posted in the toilets, and park employees live nearby. The campgrounds are rarely full—in fact, Canyon View closes during the off-season because of lack of use. If you come when only Sunset View is open, check out site 7, which is below the road and has a nice tent spot; site 15, which is very private at the price of a little hill climb; or site 16, which is nicely screened. The weather can turn cold and snowy in the winter, and no open campfires are permitted in either campground.

The Park Service offers daily, free ranger-led hikes to the 125-room alcove at Betatakin (ledge house, also known as *Talastima* in Hopi). Allow three to five hours for this 5-mile round-trip hike. The less ambitious can spot Betatakin from the overlook 0.5 miles down the paved Sandal Trail. Along the path, interpretive signs teach you the Navajo and Hopi names of native plants and their traditional uses. An additional 0.8 miles down the steep Aspen Trail allows you a glimpse into a rare pocket of forest lush with aspen and Douglas fir. If

KEY INFORMATION

ADDRESS:	Navajo National Monument HC-71 Box 3 Tonalea, AZ 86044
OPERATED BY:	National Park Service
INFORMATION:	(928) 672-2700, www.nps.gov/ nava
OPEN:	April 1– September 30
SITES:	14
EACH SITE:	Picnic table, standing grill
ASSIGNMENT:	First come, first served; no reservations
REGISTRATION:	None required
FACILITIES:	Portable toilets, group sites
PARKING:	At campsites
FEE:	None; donations accepted
ELEVATION:	7,300 feet
RESTRICTIONS:	*Pets:* On leash only; not allowed on trails *Fires:* No wood fires *Alcohol:* Prohibited *Vehicles:* 28-foot length limit *Other:* 7-day stay limit per calendar year; firearms prohibited

MAP

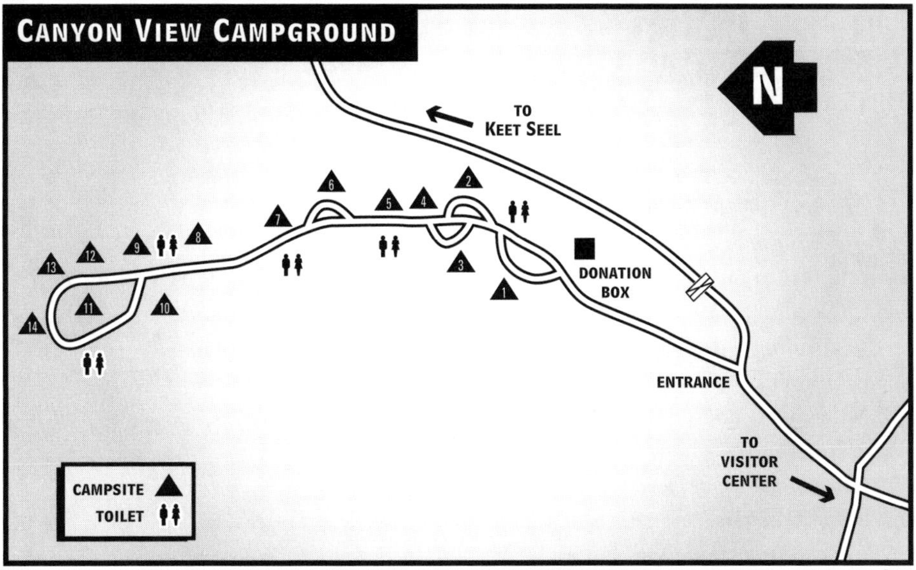
CANYON VIEW CAMPGROUND
N
TO
KEET SEEL
1
2
3
4
5
6
7
8
9
10
11
12
13
14
DONATION
BOX
ENTRANCE
TO
VISITOR
CENTER
CAMPSITE
TOILET

GETTING THERE

From Kayenta, take US 160 southwest 21 miles to AZ 564. Turn right and drive north 9 miles to the Navajo National Monument Visitor Center. Past the visitor center parking lot, turn right at the fork and drive 0.5 miles to Canyon View Campground.

you're up for a longer hike or even a backpack trip, sign up for the 17-mile round-trip hike to Keet Seel (broken pottery, *Kawestima* in Hopi), the largest and longest-inhabited of the ruins. The hike requires a backcountry permit, which is free at the visitor center. Only 20 people per day can hike to Keet Seel, so you should make reservations. The path brings you down to the riverbed, with 32 stream crossings and an occasional waterfall along the way. While you can do this as a day hike, you might prefer to backpack in and camp overnight in grasses and trees 0.25 miles from Keet Seel. At the ruin, a ranger guides you up a tall ladder and into the past, five people at a time. Inscription House (*Tsu'ovi*), the most fragile of the three, is closed to visitors.

GPS COORDINATES

Zone 12S
Easting 540877
Northing 4059798
North 36° 40' 58.56"
West 110° 32' 32.94"

5
WINDY POINT
RECREATION SITE

MOST PEOPLE WHO MAKE THE DRIVE from Kingman to Las Vegas don't pay much attention to the rugged, forlorn-looking hills to the east. The Cerbat Mountains have their secrets, however, including wild horses, several ghost towns (one alive and well), and two Bureau of Land Management (BLM) campgrounds. To get there, leave US 93 at Big Wash Road and begin the climb up into the mountains. This is the Mojave Desert, whose barren expanses make the Sonoran Desert with its trademark saguaros seem green by comparison. It seems surprising to find anything along this road, but as you switchback higher, the air cools and pinyon and juniper appear.

Tiny Packsaddle is the first campground you come to, where the road crosses the spine of the Cerbats. There are four sites here—two on each side of the road—tucked among the junipers and available at no charge. Follow the rock-lined path uphill to reach the two small sites on the right. The fire rings have been reinforced by extra rocks, which suggested to us chilly nights for previous campers. Large pinyon pines shade parts of site 1. Sites 3 and 4, across the road, are a bit larger and the ground is more level. Site 3 has a generous tent area hidden among the trees and an upright grill. Packsaddle might offer a bit more shelter when gales roar over the ridge, but we recommend that you sign in at the BLM logbook and continue the additional 1.5 miles to Windy Point.

The road takes you along the ridgeline and out to Windy Point, where seven sites sit on a spur overlooking the town of Chloride. The campground is arranged in a loop with all of the sites radiating out from the center. Ample room exists between the sites, and each one has a great view of the valley below and very little view of its neighbors. The pinyon and juniper are joined here by manzanita and scrub live oak. Windy

> *Each site has a great view of the valley below and very little view of its neighbors.*

RATINGS

Beauty: ✿ ✿ ✿ ✿
Privacy: ✿ ✿ ✿ ✿
Spaciousness: ✿ ✿ ✿ ✿ ✿
Quiet: ✿ ✿ ✿ ✿ ✿
Security: ✿ ✿ ✿
Cleanliness: ✿ ✿ ✿

KEY INFORMATION

ADDRESS: Kingman Field Office
2755 Mission Blvd.
Kingman, AZ 86401

OPERATED BY: Bureau of Land Management

INFORMATION: (928) 718-3700, www.blm.gov/az/outrec/camping/camping.htm

OPEN: Year-round

SITES: 7

EACH SITE: Picnic table, fire ring

ASSIGNMENT: First come, first served; no reservations

REGISTRATION: On-site self-registration

FACILITIES: Vault toilets

PARKING: At campsites

FEE: $4

ELEVATION: 6,200 feet

RESTRICTIONS: *Pets:* On leash only
Fires: In fire rings only
Alcohol: Permitted
Vehicles: Travel trailers are not recommended
Other: 14-day stay limit; discharging of firearms prohibited; no drinking water available

Point is aptly named, so be sure to bring your windbreaker and secure your tent well. We found the campground clean and well maintained, except that the wind had knocked over two of the trash cans and was liberally redistributing their contents.

Site 1, nestled against a mound of boulders, sees a bit of the road but none of the rest of the campground. It offers a large, sandy tent area and a pinyon-shaded picnic table. Site 2 is compact, but doesn't feel it, with pinyons providing a touch of shade. One of the tentable areas at site 3 sits right on the edge of a terrific view; with two tables and several tent spots, this would be a good site for a larger family. Site 4 also features some sheltering boulders—no shade, but plenty of privacy. A short trail from site 5 leads out to a rocky outcrop. The picnic table and fire pit at site 6 are below the level of the parking tab, between a large pinyon and a juniper, with a large, flat tent area open to the afternoon sun and a view of Cherum Peak. Site 7 is similar, a bit roomier but with less shade. The tent pad faces west, with views stretching for miles.

Spend the afternoon hiking the 3-mile Cherum Peak Trail up 1,000 feet through pinyons and chaparral to the peak. From here you can see four states: Utah, Nevada, California, and Arizona. The trail was forged and has been maintained by volunteers as well as by the Arizona Conservation Corps, a career-building program for young adults. While hiking to the 6,983-foot summit, keep an eye out for the mustangs that roam the Cerbat Mountains. The hardy wild horses are believed to be descendants of mounts that escaped or were stolen from Spanish explorers. The BLM currently manages the herd very lightly, as the mountain lions that also thrive in this area do a good job of keeping the population in balance. Peregrine falcons nest in the cliffs and spires of the Cerbat Pinnacles, an impressive geologic formation in the Mount Tipton Wilderness that crowns the Cerbats north of Big Wash Road. There are no maintained trails in the wilderness, so you'll need topo maps and route-finding skills to hike there; the BLM will happily provide more information.

The thriving ghost town of Chloride is in the foothills of the Cerbats. Experienced drivers with high

MAP

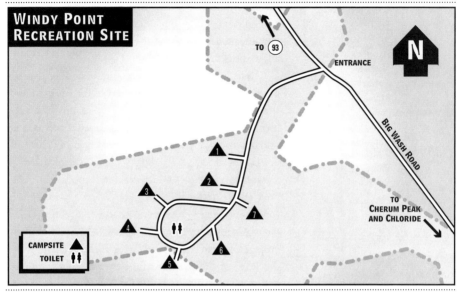

WINDY POINT
RECREATION SITE

TO ⑨③

ENTRANCE

N

BIG WASH ROAD

TO
CHERUM PEAK
AND CHLORIDE

CAMPSITE ▲
TOILET 🚻

clearance can continue from Windy Point through the remains of several mines to get to the town, or for an easier drive you can head back to the highway. Named after silver chloride that was mined in the Cerbat Mountains, Chloride was home to nearly 2,000 people at the turn of the 20th century. Today, the population is closer to 300, but many of the old buildings still stand. You can tour the town and see the oldest still-operating post office in Arizona, catch an all-female gunfight show by the Wild Roses, and view unique rock murals painted by artist Roy Purcell.

GETTING THERE

From Kingman, take US 93 northwest 18 miles to Big Wash Road. Turn right and go 10 miles to the campground entrance. Turn right into the campground.

GPS COORDINATES

Zone 11S

Easting 757939

Northing 3925252

North 35° 26' 14.34"

West 114° 9' 30.60"

6
WILD COW SPRINGS RECREATION SITE

> *It's obvious that someone has cared for this campground.*

GETTING TO WILD COW SPRINGS RECREATION SITE is part of the fun. The drive takes you up into the Hualapai Mountains, steadily climbing 3,000 feet above the Kingman Valley below. The mountains, covered in Gambel oak, ponderosa pines, and craggy granite rock, offer a nice respite during the hot summer months and a great escape year-round. The oaks blaze yellow in the fall; in winter, snow often blankets the mountains and provides smooth hills to toboggan. Spring sprinkles the forest floor with wildflowers.

Past the small community of Pine Lake, the paved road becomes dirt, very narrow, and rough, so a high-clearance vehicle with good tires is highly recommended. RVs and all but the smallest trailers definitely are not. The road climbs steadily with sheer dropoffs. You may be tempted to enjoy the splendid view of distant mountains spreading out below you, but keep your eyes on the road; no guardrail prevents that look from becoming a leap! After climbing over the ridge, you switchback down the other side of the mountain (which affords more great views) before coming to the Wild Cow Springs Recreation Site. You'll find the 18 campsites along a bumpy dirt up-and-back road. Stop at the pay station to pick up a self-pay envelope. On your right you will see a picturesque cabin that is actually the first set of vault toilets. The rest of the toilets aren't as fancy, but it's obvious that someone has cared for this campground, adding a little desert landscaping and other decorative touches.

Site 1, a small site located just off the road next to the group area, is immediately on your left. The group area is available first come, first served, costs $15 instead of $5, and offers five picnic tables, a large upright grill, and a fire ring. Site 2 is large, with a cleared, slightly raised tenting spot next to the road but sheltered by lots

RATINGS

Beauty: ✿ ✿ ✿ ✿
Privacy: ✿ ✿ ✿
Spaciousness: ✿ ✿ ✿
Quiet: ✿ ✿ ✿
Security: ✿ ✿ ✿
Cleanliness: ✿ ✿ ✿ ✿

of underbrush. The site, which has a lot of room between the picnic table and fire ring, is within easy walking distance of the toilet chalet. The Civilian Conservation Corps (CCC) built the campground in the 1930s, and most of the sites are nicely leveled and bordered by stones.

In the parking tab next to site 2, posts point out the hiking trail, lined by stones, that travels between the sites. Take this trail to get to walk-in sites 3 through 6, in the oaks across the canyon. You must cross the creek bed in order to get to these sites, which could be tricky after dark or after heavy rainfall or snowmelt. The bed forms a small-but-steep ravine, and when the creek is flowing, a waterfall cascades down the rocks near site 6. Site 7 is a handicap-accessible site right off the road with a paved path to the nearby toilets. Site 8 requires a short walk-in and is surrounded by boulders. Your picnic table here is precariously close to the edge of the ravine, but the site is nicely secluded and screened by oak trees. Sites 9 through 12 are on the opposite side of the road and all except 11 require a short uphill hike on paths hidden behind brush and oak. Sites 13 through 17 sit closer together on the ravine side of the road. These sites tend to be more popular with pop-up trailers or truck campers since the parking tabs are wider and flatter.

If you don't have a high-clearance vehicle or would like to stay somewhere more developed, stop at Hualapai Mountain Park instead of heading down past Pine Lake. This Mohave County park offers 70 campsites among ponderosa pines, large granite boulders, and rustic rental cabins. Folks with RVs should consider staying here at the small RV park instead of trying to make it down the road to Wild Cow Springs. Also near Pine Lake is the Hualapai Mountain Resort, which offers lodging and a great place to watch the elk as you dine.

From the Hualapai Mountain Park, a $5 day-use fee allows you to hike, bike, or horseback ride the 10 miles of trails in a trail system originally built by the CCC. Paths lead up to Aspen Peak (7,950 feet), Hayden Peak (8,250 feet), and Hualapai Peak (8,250 feet). Also nearby is the Wabayuma Peak Wilderness, with a trail leading to its 7,601-foot summit. High clearance and

KEY INFORMATION

ADDRESS:	Kingman Field Office 2755 Mission Blvd. Kingman, AZ 86401
OPERATED BY:	Bureau of Land Management
INFORMATION:	(928) 718-3700, www.blm.gov/az/ outrec/camping/ camping.htm
OPEN:	Year-round if accessible
SITES:	18
EACH SITE:	Picnic table, fire ring
ASSIGNMENT:	First come, first served; no reservations
REGISTRATION:	On-site self-registration
FACILITIES:	Vault toilets; group sites; handicap-accessible sites
PARKING:	At campsites
FEE:	$5, $15 for group site
ELEVATION:	6,200 feet
RESTRICTIONS:	*Pets:* On leash only *Fires:* In fire rings only *Alcohol:* Permitted *Vehicles:* 20-foot length limit; high clearance recommended; RVs and trailers not recommended *Other:* 14-day stay limit; discharging of firearms prohibited; no drinking water available

MAP

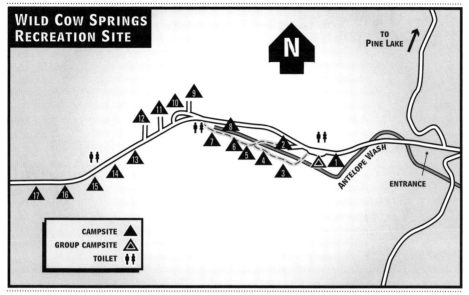

GETTING THERE

From Kingman, take Huala-pai Mountain Road southeast 14 miles to the small com-munity of Pine Lake. Turn right at Flag Mine Road and go 4 miles to Wild Cow Springs Recreation Site.

four-wheel drive is recommended to access the wilder-ness. There are also several ATV trails around Wild Cow Springs and the Pine Flat community.

If you have time, take a side trip to the historic mining town of Oatman, just 28 miles southwest of Kingman on the Historic Route 66. The drive is a National Scenic Byway. Oatman, now a thriving tourist town with restaurants and gift shops, is best known for its "wild" burros—descendents of the burros that the miners owned.

GPS COORDINATES

Zone 12S
Easting 238345
Northing 3883971
North 35° 3' 52.50"
West 113° 52' 09.30

7
DOGTOWN LAKE
CAMPGROUND

SITUATED ON OLD ROUTE 66, the city of Williams survived the arrival of the interstate and thrives on tourism in the Western theme, with steakhouses galore and gunfights staged on Main Street every summer evening. Cowboys, both live and animatronic, can be found singin', gun slingin', and even stilt-walkin' through the crowds passing by the antiques stores, gift shops, restaurants, and plenty of saloons. If cowboys prove too tame for you, grizzled mountain men follow the tradition of the town's namesake. Pioneer and trapper William Sherley Williams, often affectionately called "Old Bill," traveled through the area in the early 1800s. The Bill Williams Mountain Men celebrate the pioneer spirit of Old Bill during the annual Rendezvous Days, whose centerpiece is a 200-mile charity horseback ride from Williams to Phoenix, with riders dressed in fur, buckskins, and an impressive array of beards.

> *Enjoy the cool temperatures and tall pine forests here.*

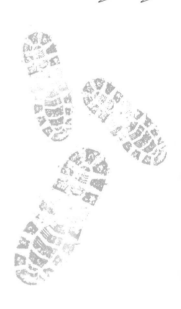

What first brought the mountain men and ranchers and then the lumbermen and railways to Williams were the trees. The Williams area shares Flagstaff's cool temperatures and tall pine forests, making it a haven for wildlife and a rich resource for early settlers. Seven lakes and reservoirs dot this area of the Kaibab National Forest, along with several campgrounds. Officials permit dispersed camping in the national forest, as long as you camp at least 0.25 miles from any water source. Some areas see very heavy use, and in the summer you'll find RVs and ATVs scattered throughout the woods.

Our favorite campground is Dogtown Lake, which is close enough to downtown Williams to partake in the festivities, yet far enough away to enjoy a peaceful evening by the campfire. The "dog" of the name is the prairie dog, whose tunnels once honeycombed this area. They're still here, as well as mule deer, skunks, porcupine, and the tassel-eared Abert's squirrel, and

RATINGS

Beauty: ✿ ✿ ✿
Privacy: ✿ ✿ ✿
Spaciousness: ✿ ✿ ✿ ✿
Quiet: ✿ ✿ ✿
Security: ✿ ✿ ✿ ✿
Cleanliness: ✿ ✿ ✿ ✿ ✿

ADDRESS:	Williams Ranger District
	742 S. Clover Rd.
	Williams, AZ
	86046
OPERATED BY:	Kaibab National Forest
INFORMATION:	(928) 635-5600, www.fs.fed.us/r3/kai
OPEN:	Full services May 1–October 1, depending on weather and roads
SITES:	54
EACH SITE:	Picnic table, fire ring
ASSIGNMENT:	First come, first served; reservations available for group sites
REGISTRATION:	On-site self-registration
FACILITIES:	Vault toilets, water spigots, recycling, picnic area, day-use ramadas, boat launch, dump station, firewood, nature trail, handicap-accessible sites
PARKING:	At campsites
FEE:	$12, $6 additional vehicle, $17 double site
ELEVATION:	7,000 feet
RESTRICTIONS:	*Pets:* On leash only *Fires:* In fire rings *Alcohol:* Permitted *Vehicles:* 35-foot limit *Other:* Swimming prohibited; 8-horsepower boat motor limit; 14-day stay limit; horses prohibited

the lake attracts plenty of waterfowl and other birds. Graded all-weather roads lead to the campground, which has a dump station but no hookups. More tent campers than RVs use the campground, and as the host told us, it's mostly hikers, hunters, and fishermen—early to bed and early to rise.

In 2003 the campground was extensively renovated for accessibility. Campers will now find clearly defined and level sites and tent pads, picnic tables with extra length on each end to accommodate wheelchairs, and sites specifically marked for handicapped campers, with paved parking tabs and standing grills.

The campground is laid out in three loops. Loops A and B are comparable, with pull-in sites on the inside and pull-through sites along the outside. Groups of up to 80 people can use loop C, but if you need just a little more room, you'll find two double sites on both the A and B loops: A5, A13, B30, and B43 (add $5). Because this is mature ponderosa forest, no underbrush screens the sites, but they are well separated. You can easily walk from the campground to the lake, but only sites A27 and A29 offer much of a lake view, and that's across the boat-ramp parking lot. On the opposite side of the campground, sites B32, B33, and B35 overlook a slope to a grassy meadow, great for bird-watching or wildlife-spotting.

The day-use area on the opposite side of the lake from the campground provides picnic tables and rental ramadas for groups. Rainbow, brown, cutthroat, and brook trout, plus catfish and crappie are stocked in the lake. Many folks simply fish from the grassy shoreline, but small boats are welcome. Swimming, however, is not permitted.

Near the boat launch you can pick up a brochure for the Ponderosa Trail, which winds its way around the area in a 1-mile self-guided nature loop. From here, you can also continue to the trail that leads you to the top of Davenport Hill, climbing nearly 800 feet in 2.5 miles. If the high altitude gets to you, enjoy the short, 1.8-mile hike around the lake instead, and admire the view of Bill Williams Mountain rising above the pines.

South of Williams lies the undeveloped gem of Sycamore Canyon. This stunning wilderness canyon

MAP

DOGTOWN LAKE CAMPGROUND

WATER ACCESS	
TOILET	
WHEELCHAIR ACCESSIBLE	
BOAT RAMP	
DUMPSITE	
GROUP AREA	

DOGTOWN LAKE

LOOP A
SITES
1–29

LOOP B
SITES
30–54

INFORMATION

INFORMATION/
FEE STATION

LOOP C
SITES
55–60

FR-132

shares the famous red rock of Sedona but is far less accessible and nearly unknown. To reach an overlook, continue down Forest Road 173 from Williams to FR 110, past Whitehorse Lake. Contact the Forest Service to find out more about the hiking trails along the rim and in the canyon itself.

To the north, of course, there's another small attraction; Williams has actually trademarked the motto "Gateway to the Grand Canyon." The Atchison, Topeka and Santa Fe Railroad Company began carrying passengers from here to the Grand Canyon in 1901, finally closing the line in 1968. In 1989, retired entrepreneurs Max and Thelma Biegert brought the line back to life, and today the Grand Canyon Railway is one of the main tourist attractions in Williams. The 2-hour-and-15-minute ride takes passengers from downtown Williams directly to Grand Canyon Village, reducing traffic and environmental impact in the park. Choose your style, from Pullman coach to luxurious parlor, or even ride atop the train in a glass-domed observation car. Wandering cowboy minstrels, fully stocked bars, and of course, a train robbery highlight the trip.

GETTING THERE

From Williams, take Fourth Street (FR 173-Perkinsville Road) south 3.5 miles to FR 140. Turn left and continue east 3 miles to FR 132. Turn left and drive north 0.75 miles to the campground.

GPS COORDINATES

Zone 12S

Easting 397464

Northing 3896628

North 35° 12' 26.76"

West 112° 7' 35.34"

8
FREIDLEIN PRAIRIE DISPERSED SITES

> *"The site sits at the ferny border of a stand of aspens overlooking a grassy meadow."*

FREIDLEIN PRAIRIE ROAD (Forest Road 522) climbs along the southern flank of the San Francisco Mountains above Flagstaff, through a dense mixed-conifer/aspen forest dotted with small clearings. Freidlein Prairie itself (sometimes spelled Friedlein or even Friedlund) is an irregular patch of aspen-rimmed grassland that, especially in fall when the trees blaze with gold, can easily be seen from town. Wildflowers abound in season, and elk and mule deer graze here throughout the year. This beautiful spot in the Coconino National Forest may have been named for an Arizona pioneer family: in 1894, the local newspaper mentioned the theft of a horse from the Friedlein brothers, as well as one Will Friedlein's successful duck-hunting trip to Mormon Lake.

Dispersed camping is allowed through most of Arizona's national forests, providing some of the state's most beautiful and serene camping experiences. In areas of very heavy human impact such as the Flagstaff urban-wildland interface, however, the Forest Service sometimes uses "designated dispersed" campsites to reduce fire risk and damage to the land. In 2001 an abandoned campfire off the Freidlein Prairie Road started the 1,300-acre Leroux fire, spurring the creation of 14 designated sites, a change meant to protect both the fragile forest and your backwoods experience. A numbered fiberglass post by the road marks each site, and another sign, "Camp within 50' of this post," defines the campsite itself. While there are no picnic tables or porta-pots, you'll find parking, a tent area, and a fire ring at every site. The beginning and end of the designated camping area are also signed.

The first two sites are fairly close to FR 516, also known as the Snowbowl Road. If you don't want to go too far up the rugged road, site 3 has a nice, open feeling. Sites 4 and 5 are neighborly, but not on top of each

RATINGS

Beauty: ✿ ✿ ✿ ✿
Privacy: ✿ ✿ ✿ ✿
Spaciousness: ✿ ✿ ✿ ✿
Quiet: ✿ ✿ ✿ ✿
Security: ✿ ✿ ✿
Cleanliness: ✿ ✿ ✿

other; sites 6 and 7 should appeal to two groups camping together, since they're just separated by a small mound of boulders. While Freidlein Prairie Road is definitely unimproved, passenger cars with good ground clearance should be able to make it as far as site 9 in dry weather.

Sites 8 and 9 sit off a recently improved spur road to the south. Wildlife spotting should be terrific from site 8, which sits at the ferny border of a stand of aspens overlooking a grassy meadow. Site 9 is among ponderosa pines at the very edge of the designated camping area. It's close to the road, but you'll see more saucy Steller's jays than passing vehicles.

Back on the main road, the landscape gets rockier. Freidlein Prairie is actually a well-known bouldering spot, with at least one published guide to the best climbs. It's a few minutes' drive to reach shallow site 10. Site 11, which is large and suitable for a group, offers several good tent spots. Sites 12 and 13 are also nice, but our pick for beauty is site 14, among lichen-covered boulders and bright-green ferns. Note that sites 10 through 14 are closed March 1 to August 31—the nesting season of the Mexican spotted owl. Any traditional nesting area may be important to the survival of this endangered species, so please respect the closure.

With no services available in the Freidlein Prairie area, pack-in/pack-out and leave-no-trace practices are encouraged. With any luck, the camper before you had good wilderness ethics, but if not, remember that an extra trash bag and five generous minutes on your part can transform a campsite for yourself and those who follow you. Keep in mind this is bear country, so be bear-safe.

Elevation along the road ranges from 7,900 to 8,600 feet, with cool summer days and the possibility of cold nights. You're near Arizona Snowbowl here, one of the state's prime ski areas, and you can expect wintry weather anytime from early fall to late spring. In the winter, Snowbowl maintains FR 516—the primary access to Freidlein Prairie Road—but the ski area's personnel only plow on weekends when the ski area is open. If you're hardy and ready to try winter camping here, check the Snowbowl and Coconino National

KEY INFORMATION

ADDRESS:	Peaks Ranger District 5075 N. Hwy. 89 Flagstaff, AZ 86004
OPERATED BY:	Coconino National Forest
INFORMATION:	(928) 526-0866, www.fs.fed.us/r3/ Coconino
OPEN:	Year-round; sites 10–14 closed March 1– August 31
SITES:	14
EACH SITE:	Fire ring
ASSIGNMENT:	First come, first served; no reservations
REGISTRATION:	None required
FACILITIES:	None
PARKING:	At campsites
FEE:	Free
ELEVATION:	7,900–8,600 feet
RESTRICTIONS:	*Pets:* On leash only *Fires:* In fire rings only *Alcohol:* Permitted *Vehicles:* RVs and trailers not recommended; motorized/mechanized vehicles not permitted in the Kachina Peaks Wilderness. *Other:* 14-day stay limit; pack in/ pack out; no drinking water available; bear country food-storage restrictions

MAP

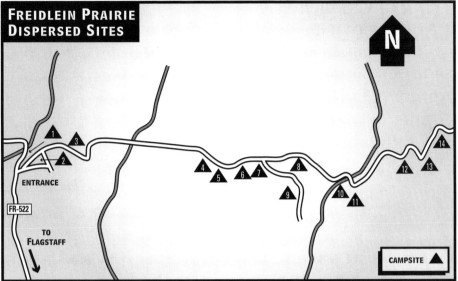

FREIDLEIN PRAIRIE DISPERSED SITES

ENTRANCE

FR-522

TO FLAGSTAFF

CAMPSITE ▲

GETTING THERE

From Flagstaff, take US 180 northwest to Snowbowl Road. Turn right and drive north 2.4 miles to FR 522. Turn right into dispersed area.

GPS COORDINATES

Zone 12S
Easting 435740
Northing 3905564
North 35° 17' 28.36"
West 111° 42' 24.18"

Forest Web sites to assess conditions. You'll need a free winter backcountry permit (available at the ski area if open or from the Peaks Ranger Station) for winter camping and snow play in the Kachina Peaks Wilderness area.

You can find summer fun at Snowbowl, as well, with daily scenic lift rides up Agassiz Peak and ranger talks at the top on weekends. Have a deli-style lunch at the Peak Side Cafe in the Agassiz Lodge, then head out for a hike. You can use Snowbowl as the jumping-off point for some great hikes in the Kachina Peaks Wilderness, including a 4.5-mile, 3,300-foot climb to the top of Humphreys Peak (Arizona's highest at 12,633 feet) and the Kachina Trail, a more moderate 7-mile ramble across the slopes of the ancient volcano, which terminates at the end of FR 522.

For more information about Flagstaff's charms and area attractions, see profile 9, Lockett Meadow Campground.

9
LOCKETT MEADOW CAMPGROUND

APPROACHING FLAGSTAFF FROM ANY DIREC-
TION, the first things you'll notice are the San
Francisco Peaks. Volcanic upheaval created
this range, and after 1 million years of erosion, these
are still Arizona's highest mountains. For centuries
the peaks, frequently snow-capped or shrouded in
rain clouds, have held spiritual significance for Native
Americans. They form the Sacred Mountain of the
West and the boundary of the Navajo Nation. They're
also visible from the mesas of the Hopi, who believe
that the Kachina spirits call these mountains home.
The Kachina Peaks Wilderness encompasses the heart
of this ancient volcano.

On the edge of this wilderness, nestled high on
the eastern slopes, is the alpine haven of Lockett
Meadow Campground. The narrow unpaved road
winds up the mountain, revealing magnificent views
past the cinder cones and lava fields of Sunset Crater
National Monument and out to the Painted Desert.
This challenging route is usually passable by passenger
cars in dry weather, but is definitely not recommended
for RVs or trailers. At its end, towering Douglas fir,
ponderosa pines, and quaking aspens surround several
acres of upland prairie grasses, once summer grazing
for the sheep of homesteader Henry Claiborne Lockett.
In spring and summer the meadow is spangled with
wildflowers, and in late September the changing aspens
splash the mountainsides with bright gold. Stand qui-
etly at sunrise or sunset and you may see foraging elk,
mule deer, porcupine, or even a black bear. Listen for
voices of the numerous native and migratory birds. The
variety of plant and animal life found in these mountains inspired pioneering biologist C. Hart Merriam to
develop the ecological concept of life zones.

Lockett Meadow is the only campground this
high in the peaks, and it's best to arrive early—the 17
campsites cannot be reserved, and dispersed camping

> *In spring and summer
> the meadow is spangled
> with wildflowers, and
> in late September the
> changing aspens splash
> the mountainsides with
> bright gold.*

RATINGS

Beauty: ✪ ✪ ✪ ✪ ✪
Privacy: ✪ ✪ ✪ ✪
Spaciousness: ✪ ✪ ✪ ✪
Quiet: ✪ ✪ ✪ ✪
Security: ✪ ✪ ✪ ✪
Cleanliness: ✪ ✪ ✪ ✪ ✪

KEY INFORMATION

ADDRESS: Peaks Ranger District
5075 N. Hwy. 89
Flagstaff, AZ 86004

OPERATED BY: Coconino National Forest

INFORMATION: (928) 526-0866,
www.fs.fed.us/r3/
Coconino

OPEN: Mid-May to mid-October

SITES: 17

EACH SITE: Picnic table, fire ring

ASSIGNMENT: First come, first served;
no reservations

REGISTRATION: On-site self-registration

FACILITIES: Vault toilets

PARKING: At campsites, at trailhead

FEE: $10 per night, $5 per day use

ELEVATION: 8,600 feet

RESTRICTIONS: *Pets:* On leash only
Fires: In fire rings only
Alcohol: Permitted
Vehicles: RVs and trailers not recommended; 2 vehicles per site; ATVs or motorbikes prohibited except to and from campground; mountain bikes prohibited in wilderness
Other: 14-day stay limit; 8 people per site; bear country food-storage restrictions; firearms prohibited; horses prohibited

is not permitted near the meadow. The high elevation means you'll enjoy comfortable temperatures all summer, but come prepared for chilly evenings and quickly changing mountain weather in any season. The road is closed in the winter and the campground is not maintained from October to May, but hardy souls on skis or snowshoes are welcome to use the campsites with a backcountry permit.

As you reach the campground, the road becomes one-way. The meadow itself is protected grassland closed to camping and vehicles. The campsites are outside the loop, nestled under a canopy of pale aspens and mature ponderosa pines with their vanilla-scented bark. Each site has a picnic table and a fire ring; in dry Arizona it's always a good idea to check with the Forest Service about fire restrictions. Pull in to the self-service pay station and check out site 1; it's close but nicely screened from the road, and one of the two wildlife watering holes is just through the trees. Our favorite sites are near the trailhead, but once the day-use traffic is gone, site 7 may be the most secluded in the campground. Campsites 9 through 11 provide more room for larger groups, but are also more open to the road and each other. The best views of the meadow and the second pond are from sites 13 through 16. Two sets of vault toilets serve the campground; there are no other facilities and no drinking water. You won't have a host, but the campground feels fairly secure. Though popular, Lockett Meadow still leaves you with an impression of remoteness and serenity.

The Inner Basin Trail begins its steady uphill climb at the Lockett Meadow Campground. The wide, even trail makes a pleasant 3.9-mile round-trip through the forest of the caldera. You'll top 10,000 feet, so be aware of your conditioning and pace yourself. If you're very ambitious, follow the Weatherford Trail to the Humphreys Trail, which takes you to Arizona's highest point (12,634 feet). On a clear day you may see all the way to the North Rim of the Grand Canyon. If you have less time or stamina, you can also reach Humphreys Peak by a shorter route from the Snowbowl ski area. Don't be ashamed if acclimated Flagstaff residents jog past you twice while you're still toiling up the trail.

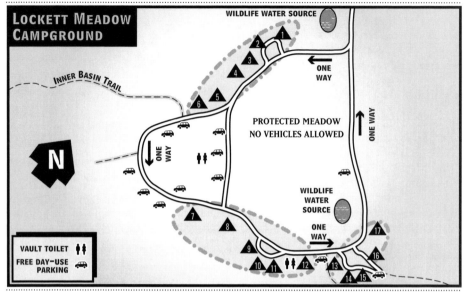

LOCKETT MEADOW CAMPGROUND

WILDLIFE WATER SOURCE

INNER BASIN TRAIL

ONE WAY

PROTECTED MEADOW
NO VEHICLES ALLOWED

ONE WAY

N

WILDLIFE
WATER
SOURCE

ONE WAY

VAULT TOILET
FREE DAY–USE PARKING

From the inner basin you can also access the strenuous Abineau/Bear Jaw loop hike, which is equally lovely but much less popular. Most of the trail system is in the Kachina Peaks Wilderness, and mountain bikes are not permitted in the fragile alpine environment. Horses, dogs, and camping are also forbidden in the inner basin to protect the mountain aquifer.

Outside the wilderness boundary, Flagstaff is a thriving community rich in natural and human history. Recreational options for all tastes and seasons include downhill and cross-country skiing at Snowbowl and the Flagstaff Nordic Center, plus plenty of mountain biking in the Coconino National Forest. Crawl through Lava River Cave for an intimate experience of volcanic geology, or stand on the doorstep of history at the ancient pueblos of Wupatki National Monument. Peer into the heavens during a star party at Lowell Observatory, originally built to map the illusory canals of Mars. Or just sit back beneath the aspens in Lockett Meadow and take it easy.

GETTING THERE

From Flagstaff, take US 89 northeast. Turn left at the forest access sign (FR 420, but the road is not signed with the road number, only the forest access sign) directly across from the turn to Sunset Crater National Monument. Continue approximately 0.5 miles to the signed intersection and turn right on FR 552. Follow the signs to the campground.

GPS COORDINATES

Zone 12S

Easting 443694

Northing 3913213

North 35° 21' 38.28"

West 111° 37' 11.16"

10
MANZANITA
CAMPGROUND

> *Perennial Oak Creek has carved this narrow, verdant passage that provides a beautiful setting for fishing, swimming, hiking, or just relaxing.*

SEDONA HAS SOMETIMES BEEN CALLED the most beautiful place in the United States. The distinctive red-rock mountains create whimsical shapes that have been named whatever the imagination sees in them—Coffeepot, Snoopy, Cathedral, and Bell. Many believe that these mountains contain vortexes of ethereal energy whose power can be felt throughout the city. Artists and New Agers flock here, and you can stroll through the many art galleries, get your tarot cards read, have a past-life regression, or join a vortex hiking tour. Upscale boutiques rub shoulders with shops selling everything from Harley gear to energy crystals.

The stunning scenery makes for great outdoor experiences. Enjoy the surroundings on a Pink Jeep tour of the four-by-four trails, hike in the serene Secret Mountain Wilderness, or watch the sunset from your resort balcony. One of Sedona's major draws is Oak Creek Canyon. Perennial Oak Creek has carved this narrow, verdant passage that provides a beautiful setting for fishing, swimming, hiking, or just relaxing. Of the four campgrounds along Oak Creek Canyon, Manzanita is the closest to the creek. Because of its popularity, try to make a reservation ahead of time online or by phone. That way, you're not only guaranteed a spot, it'll be one of the best sites in the campground; only sites 9 through 19 are reservable and these lie right along the creek bed.

Both the north and south entrances from AZ 89A lead down to the self-service pay station and the campground host. If you have a reservation, you may continue to your site. If you're hoping for a first-come, first-served site, your best bet is to come early in the morning or on a weekday. Sites 1 through 3 are close together in the middle of the campground loop and don't offer any privacy, and sites 6 and 7 are also quite

RATINGS

Beauty: ✿ ✿ ✿ ✿
Privacy: ✿ ✿
Spaciousness: ✿ ✿ ✿
Quiet: ✿ ✿ ✿
Security: ✿ ✿ ✿ ✿
Cleanliness: ✿ ✿ ✿ ✿ ✿

open and close to the road. Raised above the campground on a leveled shelf, site 5 is a nice, compact site with its back to the highway. Site 4, at the end of the loop, sits a little apart from its neighbors, but for privacy and spaciousness, take 19. If you have a group, sites 9 and 10 are close together past the host in site 8, and they almost have a stretch of the creek to themselves. You'll need to be able to parallel park for sites 11 through 15, but the sites are reasonably spaced. The tight loop road discourages trailers and RVs; expect to pay an extra $7 fee if you come with two vehicles. You can take a shower farther north at the much-larger Cave Spring Campground; just let the staff at the entry station know you're camped at Manzanita, and they'll sell you a token.

AZ 89A snakes up the narrow canyon, making some traffic noise unavoidable. The sound of the creek lulls you to sleep anyway, and the campground itself is very quiet. The creek flow depends on rainfall and snowmelt, and on rare occasions has risen over the stone retaining walls and swirled around the picnic tables. On the south side of the campground, past sites 9 and 10, the creek opens up to form a large swimming hole where a rickety rope swing hangs high above the water. A trail leads from the north end of the campground and passes the foundations of an old homestead with feral apple trees in the front garden. The campground is in a stand of ponderosa pines, box elders, and Arizona ash that, along with the high red cliffs, provide ample shade.

Look for the large sacred datura blooming near the entrance. Also called jimsonweed or thornapple, its large, white blossoms open during the night and close the following morning. This member of the nightshade family has been used by Native Americans for inducing trances, but is often fatal for people who experiment with its hallucinogenic properties.

South of the campground is Grasshopper Point, a great swimming hole created by Oak Creek at the base of a cliff. Just 0.75 miles north of the campground is Slide Rock State Park, where the smooth, slick rock of the creek bottom has created a natural slide popular with families. Thrill seekers also enjoy jumping from

KEY INFORMATION

ADDRESS:	Red Rock Ranger District P.O. Box 20249 Sedona, AZ 86341
OPERATED BY:	Coconino National Forest
INFORMATION:	(928) 282-4119, www.fs.fed.us/r3/coconino
OPEN:	Year-round
SITES:	19
EACH SITE:	Picnic table, fire ring
ASSIGNMENT:	First come, first served; reservations available for sites 9–19, 2 days in advance
REGISTRATION:	Online, with camp host, on-site self-registration
FACILITIES:	Vault toilets, water spigots, pay phone, campground host, firewood
PARKING:	At campsites
FEE:	$18 (plus $9 reservation fee if purchased online), $7 additional vehicle, $7 day-use
ELEVATION:	4,800 feet
RESTRICTIONS:	*Pets:* On leash only *Fires:* In fire rings only *Alcohol:* Permitted *Vehicles:* RVs or trailers prohibited; ATVs prohibited *Other:* 7-day stay limit; firearms prohibited

MAP

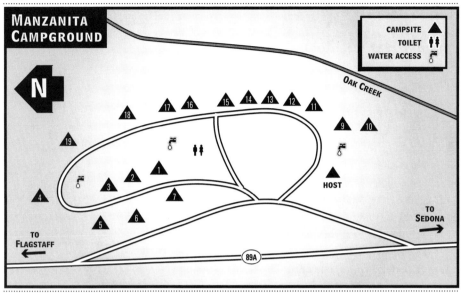

GETTING THERE

From Sedona, take AZ 89A north 6 miles. Turn right into the campground.

the surrounding boulders into the creek's cool pools. An apple orchard from the park's former life as a farmstead still bears fruit today.

A little farther north is Call of the Canyon day-use area, named after the Zane Grey novel set here, and the trailhead for the West Fork Trail, the most popular trail in the Coconino National Forest. This scenic path crosses the stream several times and is rich in wildlife and beautifully weathered rock. The first 3 miles are the most heavily used, but if you enjoy bouldering and the occasional swim, you can hike all 14 miles of the canyon. You'll need to purchase a Red Rock Pass to use any of the National Forest land in the Sedona area, including hiking trails, picnic areas, and the many ruins and heritage sites.

GPS COORDINATES

Zone 12S
Easting 431980
Northing 3866171
North 34° 56' 08.70"
West 111° 44' 41.34"

11
KINNIKINICK LAKE CAMPGROUND

AS THE TEMPERATURES IN THE DESERT valleys creep up into the triple digits, people start flocking to Arizona's high country. The Mormon Lake area is a popular summer retreat, with many small lakes and several good campgrounds lining scenic Lake Mary Road south from Flagstaff toward Payson. Our favorite of these is Kinnikinick Lake, a little gem in the pinyon-juniper grasslands.

The route from Flagstaff takes you past Upper Lake Mary, a popular spot for boating, waterskiing, fishing, and bird-watching, to Mormon Lake. This is Arizona's largest natural lake, but don't expect much fishing here, as it's often nearly dry. The resulting marshy pasture is a great place to view wildlife, so stop at the overlook and see if you can spot a bald eagle flying overhead, or elk grazing on the tall grasses. One (possibly tall) tale we've been told is that as many as 50 elk will gather in the middle of the lake bed during hunting season, as if some instinct tells them that no hunter will take a shot in the face of an impossibly soggy retrieval.

Near the south end of Mormon Lake, turn east onto Forest Road 125, a well-graded dirt road that carries you onto higher ground, passing through large, grassy meadows speckled with ponderosa pines and a few oaks. Look northwest to see the San Francisco Peaks rising over the trees in the distance. This good grazing land borders the Anderson Mesa Wildlife Protection Area, so keep an eye out for elk, mule deer, antelope, and cattle as you drive past Mud Lake, which often lives up to its name. Kinnikinick gets its own name from the bearberry shrub (*Arctostaphylos uva-ursi*), a widespread relative of the manzanita. In Algonquin, the term means mixture: the leaves were often mixed in with tobacco and smoked or burned by Native Americans.

As you pull into the campground, take a right at the fork in the road and drive down to the boat ramp,

> *If you intend to fish or would like to wake up to the sun rising over the lake, no need to go any farther.*

RATINGS

Beauty: ✩ ✩ ✩ ✩
Privacy: ✩ ✩ ✩
Spaciousness: ✩ ✩ ✩
Quiet: ✩ ✩ ✩
Security: ✩ ✩ ✩ ✩
Cleanliness: ✩ ✩ ✩ ✩

KEY INFORMATION

ADDRESS:	Mormon Lake Ranger District 4373 South Lake Mary Road Flagstaff, AZ 86001
OPERATED BY:	Coconino National Forest
INFORMATION:	(928) 774-1147, www.fs.fed.us/r3/coconino
OPEN:	Year-round if accessible; full services mid-May–October 1
SITES:	13
EACH SITE:	Picnic table, fire ring
ASSIGNMENT:	First come, first served; no reservations
REGISTRATION:	With camp host
FACILITIES:	Vault toilets, firewood, boat ramp, campground host, day-use area
PARKING:	At campsites
FEE:	$14 per night, $7 day use, $7 second vehicle
ELEVATION:	7,000 feet
RESTRICTIONS:	*Pets:* On leash only *Fires:* Permitted in fire rings only *Alcohol:* Permitted *Vehicles:* 22-foot length limit; 2 vehicles per site; motorbikes restricted to entering and exiting campsite *Other:* 14-day stay limit; 8 people per site; 10-horsepower boat-motor size limit; horses prohibited; no drinking water available

day-use area, and sites 1 and 2. If you intend to fish or would like to wake up to the sun rising over the lake, no need to go any farther. These two sites are the closest to the water and are away from the others, so once the day-use area clears out, you should have a quiet evening.

If you'd prefer to be farther away from early-rising fishermen, turn around and head down the other tine of the fork. The campground is set on a slight hill, so most of the sites command some view of the lake. All contain a picnic table and a steel fire ring with a grill, and most have a cleared, leveled tent area. Campground hosts, who live here from mid-May through the end of September, take site number 5. Taller junipers, a few pines, and a bit more shade distinguish sites 8 through 11. There is no unlucky 13 here, so it's site 14 at the end of the loop, with no close neighbors and a great view of the lake. The sites are best suited for tent camping, but a handful will accommodate small RVs.

Man-made Kinnikinick Lake was dammed to provide water for nearby ranches and a reservoir for forest firefighters. The lake, while small, is frequently stocked with brook, brown, and rainbow trout, so bring your fishing pole and canoe or small boat (as long as the motor is less than 10 horsepower). Come here for great bird-watching, particularly during migrations. If you should see an osprey drop from the sky and splash up with a fish, look for the bird to turn the catch in its talons in flight so that it faces aerodynamically forward. During spring you may see western grebes courting with their long, swanlike necks, and look for coots and other waterfowl year-round. Mountain bluebirds are everywhere, and in the early-morning hours you won't be able to miss the cascading, liquid call of the meadowlark. You may also see less-attractive fliers; bring bug spray for spring's no-see-um gnats. You won't find signed trails at Kinnikinick, but ask the campground host about hiking to a prehistoric site in the area. Hunters and avid fishermen can use the campground in the off-season, but without the comfort of facilities. In bad winter weather, the road may be closed.

If you get sick of your camp cooking, head over to Mormon Lake Lodge at Mormon Lake Village. The lodge, open since 1924, has a restaurant and a general

MAP

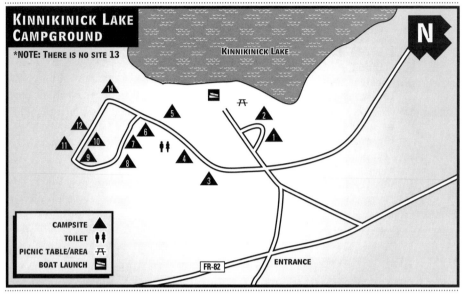

KINNIKINICK LAKE CAMPGROUND

*NOTE: THERE IS NO SITE 13

KINNIKINICK LAKE

N

CAMPSITE ▲
TOILET ♀♂
PICNIC TABLE/AREA 𐐨
BOAT LAUNCH ⊟

FR-82   ENTRANCE

store. A catastrophic fire burned the original lodge to the ground in 1974, but local ranchers rebuilt it, and the interior walls still display their cattle brands. Western literature buffs will find a nice selection of Zane Grey memorabilia, as well as a plethora of game trophies. The village also offers gasoline, riding stables, rental cabins, and winter recreation, including snowmobile and cross-country ski rentals.

GETTING THERE

From Flagstaff, take Lake Mary Road (FR 3) south 30 miles to FR 125. Turn left and drive east 5.5 miles to FR 82. Turn right and continue southeast 4 miles to campground.

GPS COORDINATES

Zone 12S

Easting 471409

Northing 3861368

North 34° 53' 39.54"

West 111° 18' 46.50"

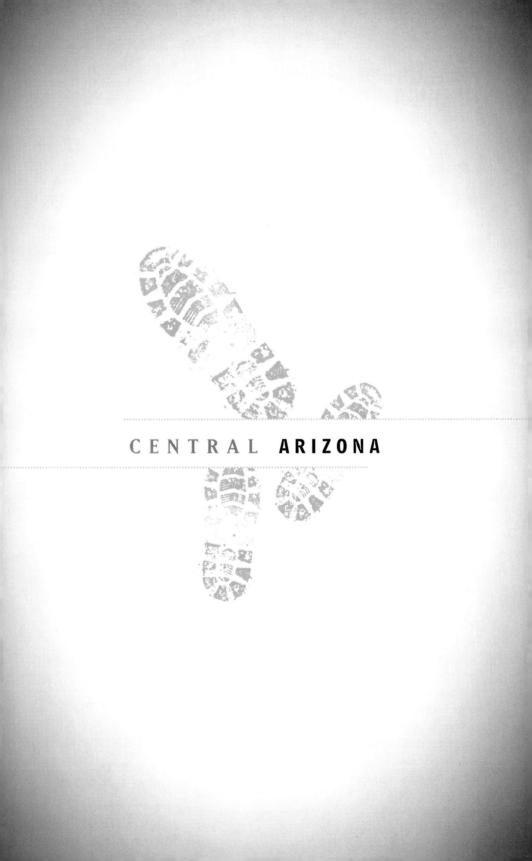

CENTRAL **ARIZONA**

12
MINGUS MOUNTAIN
CAMPGROUND

A SINUOUS SECTION OF AZ 89A, designated the
Mingus Mountain Scenic Road, snakes its way
from Jerome across the Black Hills toward
Prescott. These hills have been mined since prehistoric times, and if you look closely, piles of telltale
tailings will reveal where fortunes were made and (far
more often) lost. Where the road passes over the hills'
summit, turn in to the picnic parking at Forest Road
104 for some interpretive tidbits. This is also your
turn for the twisting but manageable dirt road up to
Mingus Mountain. On your way, peruse the Church
Meadow Wildlife Area, where you may spot shy
pronghorn antelope grazing. Past the Methodist
church camp, you'll find Mingus Lake (formerly called
Elk Tank). Swimming and boating are prohibited on
this tiny lake, but it is stocked with rainbow trout.
There is a $2 day-use fee, as there is for the nearby
vista and picnic area.

The picnic area, still called Loop A, was once part
of the old campground, but recent renovations have
resulted in 19 new sites. Six of the older sites, loop B,
have been designated tent-only. Although these are
shady, head up the road to loop E. This loop was built
with electrical hookups and plumbing—intended as a
major upgrade—but the last few years' disastrous fire
seasons sapped the Forest Service budget, and work has
stalled. As an unintended benefit, RVs may be discouraged from braving the road up.

For now you'll need to bring your own water, and
the Forest Service encourages people to clear their own
tent area in lieu of the intended pads. Although the
ground is not ideal, the expansive mountaintop feeling
and terrific view make up for it. From sites 6, 8, 10, and
11, take your camp chair for a short stroll to the edge
and settle in to contemplate the neverending view over
the Verde Valley to the Secret Mountain Wilderness

> *Take your camp chair
> for a short stroll to the
> edge and settle in
> to contemplate the
> neverending view.*

RATINGS

Beauty: ✰ ✰ ✰ ✰
Privacy: ✰ ✰ ✰
Spaciousness: ✰ ✰ ✰ ✰ ✰
Quiet: ✰ ✰ ✰
Security: ✰ ✰ ✰
Cleanliness: ✰ ✰ ✰ ✰

ADDRESS:	Bradshaw Ranger District 344 South Cortez Street Prescott, AZ 86303
OPERATED BY:	Prescott National Forest
INFORMATION:	(928) 443-8000, www.fs.fed.us/r3/prescott
OPEN:	Managed season May 1–October 31
SITES:	25
EACH SITE:	Picnic table, fire ring, electrical hookups
ASSIGNMENT:	First come, first served; no reservations
REGISTRATION:	On-site self-registration
FACILITIES:	Vault toilets, campground host
PARKING:	At campsites
FEE:	$6; $2 day-use
ELEVATION:	7,500 feet
RESTRICTIONS:	*Pets:* On leash only *Fires:* In fire rings only *Alcohol:* Permitted *Vehicles:* 22-foot length limit *Other:* 14-day stay limit; no drinking water available; quiet hours 10 p.m.–6 a.m.; 10 people per site; checkout 2 p.m.

and the red rocks of Sedona. The best tent spots developing so far are at sites 5 and 8 through 11, although possibilities exist for all but sites 2, 6, and 13.

At 7,500 feet you'll find the temperature pleasantly cool in the summer. The wind often rises over the mountain and blows across the summit—incentive to stake your tent and one reason hang gliders love this spot. Two Arizona Hang Glider Association cliff launch points are up the road across the vista day-use area. If you prefer to keep your feet on terra firma, the campground makes a good base for exploring the region's numerous hiking trails. The View Point Trail #106 near the day-use area only *seems* to drop off the cliff, and it makes a moderate 4.25-mile loop hike when combined with North Mingus Trail #105 and #105A. It's especially beautiful in fall when the maples and oaks begin to change. Across the highway in Potato Patch Campground is Woodchute Trail, a mild 8-mile round-trip through designated wilderness to spectacular panoramic views from the north end of Woodchute Mountain.

No trip to the Black Hills is complete without a stop in what was once the "wickedest town in America" and is now the liveliest ghost town you'll ever see. Built by hard-rock miners on the 30-degree slopes of Cleopatra Hill, precarious Jerome supported one of the most successful mines in the world, generating $1 million a month at its peak. In the 1920s, 15,000 residents called it home, making it the fourth-largest city in Arizona. The miners' lives were tough; they took pleasure where they could, and the town was filled with saloons, gambling halls, opium dens, and brothels, staying wild well past the taming of the rest of the West. When the mines closed in 1953, the population dwindled to a stubborn 100-or-so folks and became a ghost town. Artists, entrepreneurs, and hippies realized they could purchase the old bordellos cheaply and, slowly, art galleries, hotels, restaurants, and shops began to open. The government designated the entire town a national historic district in 1967, and today the city is a thriving artist community and a popular tourist destination, with a permanent population of about 500. Many of the old buildings are rumored to be haunted, and locals embrace the spectral past. You can eat at the Haunted Hamburger or The

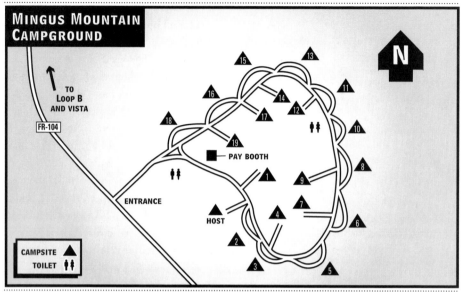

MINGUS MOUNTAIN CAMPGROUND

TO LOOP B AND VISTA

FR-104

PAY BOOTH

ENTRANCE

HOST

CAMPSITE ▲
TOILET ♦♦

Asylum or stay at the Ghost City Inn. Around Halloween, you can join the Jerome Historical Society's ghost walk or attend the annual costume ball in the community center, affectionately dubbed "Spook Hall."

Parking can be tricky on the side of a mountain, so take the first spot you see and walk. Fires and gravity have taken some of the buildings (including the town jail), but most of the remaining structures date from the turn of the last century, and only look as if they're going to give out at any second and tumble down the mountain. Stop by the Jerome Historical Society's Mine Museum and see old mining equipment, gambling goods, and photos of what Jerome looked like in its heyday.

GETTING THERE

From Jerome, take AZ 89A southwest 9 miles uphill to FR 104. Turn left and go southeast 2.5 miles to the stop sign. Turn right and head 0.5 miles to the campground. Turn left into the campground.

GPS COORDINATES

Zone 12S

Easting 397489

Northing 3839425

North 34° 41' 30.12"

West 112° 7' 09.06"

13
YAVAPAI CAMPGROUND

> *The craggy peaks of Granite Mountain rise in the distance.*

PRESCOTT BEGAN LIFE WHEN Arizona's first territorial governor set up the seat of government near the protection of Fort Whipple. It lost, regained, and lost again the title of territorial capital. Today it's one of the state's fastest-growing communities, with more people every year discovering the ideal Arizona climate in this mile-high city surrounded by lakes, mountains, and pine forests. Roll into town and you'll probably find an art fair or other event going on in the grassy square of the historic Yavapai County Courthouse in the center of downtown. Montezuma Street no longer has 40 saloons as it did in the good ol' days, but several bars keep historic "Whiskey Row" alive with nightly live music and dancing. The World's Oldest Rodeo is held in Prescott, and the broncos buck and the cowboys strut annually during the week of Independence Day.

Just 8 miles northwest of downtown, Yavapai Campground butts up against the 9,799-acre Granite Mountain Wilderness. The craggy peaks of Granite Mountain rise in the distance to 7,626 feet. Twenty-five sites are arranged in a loop among large boulders (granite, naturally), scrub oak, cliff rose, manzanita, junipers, and ponderosa pines. All of the sites are well separated from one another and screened by chaparral, and each one has a picnic table and metal fire ring with grill. A few also have an upright grill. Three double sites—2 and 3, 6 and 7, and 16 and 17—share parking tabs, and have two picnic tables and two fire pits in fairly close proximity. If the rest of the campground is full, separate parties could use these sites, but if you prefer your privacy, they should be left to large groups or families traveling together. The two handicap-accessible sites, 8 and 21, are the only ones with electrical hookups. Sites 8, 9, and 10 are all in a row and share a parking lot. Sites 14, 15, and 22 are our favorites. The picnic table

RATINGS

Beauty: ☆ ☆ ☆ ☆
Privacy: ☆ ☆ ☆ ☆
Spaciousness: ☆ ☆ ☆
Quiet: ☆ ☆ ☆
Security: ☆ ☆ ☆ ☆
Cleanliness: ☆ ☆ ☆ ☆ ☆

and fire pit at site 14 are slightly separated from the parking area in a split-level design. Site 15 is set back so that you can't see the road or any other sites—just trees, brush, and sky. A nearby boulder makes a good perch for watching the light change on Granite Mountain. Site 22 wins the award for the cutest site, with six steps leading up to the raised tent pad hidden behind a tall, slender granite monolith.

Just down the road is 5-acre Granite Basin Lake. The tiny lake is not stocked, but you can still throw out a line as an excuse just to sit a bit, and you might get a bite from a bluegill or catfish. Picnic tables and drinking water are available at the Playa Picnic Area. You'll usually find a selection of waterbirds here, including stately blue herons and contentious coots. The mountain looms across the lake, studded with enormous jagged outcrops of rock. Peregrine falcons and rock climbers are equally attracted to these rugged cliffs; if you're interested in climbing, check with the Forest Service about nesting closures and anchor rules. Near the lake you'll also find Granite Group, a reservation-only area with varying fees for up to 100 people. While Yavapai is open year-round, the group site is closed in the winter.

When you're ready to explore the network of trails around the campground, the host can provide you with a map of the Granite Basin Recreation Area. You can start your hike from the trailhead near site 11, or you can park at any of the four trailhead parking lots on the way down to the lake: Cayuse, Wekuvde, Metate, or at the boat launch. Granite Mountain Trail #261 begins at the Metate trailhead and switchbacks up through the Granite Mountain Wilderness to Vista Point Overlook at one of the peaks. From here you can look out over the lake, Chino Valley, Skull Valley, and Prescott itself. The trip to the viewpoint is a strenuous 7.7-mile round-trip, but there's plenty of great stuff to see no matter how far

KEY INFORMATION

ADDRESS:	Bradshaw Ranger District, 344 South Cortez Street, Prescott, AZ 86303
OPERATED BY:	Prescott National Forest
INFORMATION:	(928) 443-8000, www.fs.fed.us/r3/prescott
OPEN:	Year-round
SITES:	25
EACH SITE:	Picnic table, fire ring, some have an upright grill
ASSIGNMENT:	First come, first served; reservations accepted for group site
REGISTRATION:	On-site self-registration
FACILITIES:	Composting toilets, water spigots, boat ramp at Granite Basin Lake, beach, picnic area, picnic shelters, day-use area, day-use ramadas, nature trails, group sites, campground host, recycling, handicap-accessible sites
PARKING:	At campsites
FEE:	$10; $2 day-use
ELEVATION:	5,600 feet
RESTRICTIONS:	*Pets:* On leash only, not permitted in lake. *Fires:* In fire rings only. *Alcohol:* Permitted. *Vehicles:* 40-foot length limit; 2 vehicles per site; 1 RV per site. *Other:* 14-day stay limit; mountain bikes prohibited; firearms prohibited; swimming prohibited, 10 people per site; electric motors only are allowed on the lake; mechanized and motorized vehicles prohibited in wilderness; quiet hours 10 p.m.–6 a.m.; checkout 2 p.m.

MAP

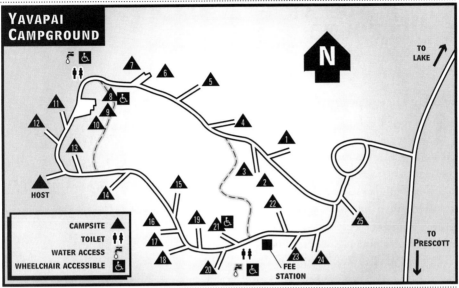

YAVAPAI CAMPGROUND

CAMPSITE
TOILET
WATER ACCESS
WHEELCHAIR ACCESSIBLE

GETTING THERE

From Prescott, take Gurley Street west to Grove Avenue. Turn right and drive north 1 mile to Iron Springs Road. Turn left and continue northwest 3 miles to FR 374. Turn right and head north 3 miles to the campground entrance. Turn left into the campground.

GPS COORDINATES

Zone 12S
Easting 358908
Northing 3830032
North 34° 36' 08.76"
West 112° 32' 19.38"

you choose to go. Loop hikes of almost any length and difficulty can be designed by linking different trails in the Granite Basin Recreation Area. You'll also find connections to additional trails for hikers, equestrians, and mountain bikers that travel throughout the Prescott area, so stock up on topo maps.

If you've brought a canoe or kayak, Granite Lake won't hold your attention long. Venture over to nearby Watson Lake in the Granite Dells area of Prescott Valley. The weird formations of piled and tumbled billion-year-old boulders that surround the lower end of the lake are a paddler's playground, and there's terrific bird-watching in the marshy shallows where Granite Creek flows in. For a varied but easy hike, try the Peavine Trail, which follows a 4.75-mile section of the old Santa Fe, Prescott & Phoenix railroad grade from the Dells out into open rangeland.

14
LOWER WOLF CREEK CAMPGROUND

THE PRESCOTT BASIN LIES TO THE SOUTH and west of the burgeoning community of Prescott and encompasses 59,000 acres of the Prescott National Forest. Mixed conifer forest covers much of the land, but stands of oak and stretches of pinyon pine and juniper woodland are also common. A wildland-urban interface area, this part of Arizona provides days of scenic drives and plenty of camping, hiking, and sightseeing opportunities.

You'll find several campgrounds in the Prescott Basin, each with its own appeal, but Lower Wolf Creek probably best suits tent campers. The campground is in a creek-carved valley, in a stand of ponderosa pine, fir, Arizona walnut, and Gambel oak. This is an old Civilian Conservation Corps camp, and the stone masonry picnic tables add rustic appeal. Boulders decorate the pine needle–strewn ground and provide extra screening in some sites. Two routes bring you here from Prescott—White Spar Road and the Senator Highway—and either is a delight. Both bring you to Forest Road 97 along well-graded dirt roads passable by passenger cars in dry weather.

Lower Wolf Creek Campground sprawls along both sides of FR 97. Pull into the south entrance and the host and sites 1 through 5 are to your left. Sites 1 and 2 are off a spur road, FR 74, which connects with Senator Highway. Here, you'll have the occasional ATV enthusiast roaring past. We liked the set-apart feel of site 3, and site 4 sits picturesquely in a nest of boulders, although FR 97 curves around closer than it first appears.

Go back past the host, and sites 8 through 16 trail to the west, following the line of the dry creek bed. If you'd like a little more solitude, head down to the sites at the end of the line. Site 14 is up a flight of stone steps from a walled, single-car pull-out and offers a spacious, sandy tent area set back from the picnic table. There's

> *Gambel oaks and walnuts become a patchwork of gold and copper.*

RATINGS

Beauty: ✿ ✿ ✿
Privacy: ✿ ✿ ✿
Spaciousness: ✿ ✿ ✿
Quiet: ✿ ✿
Security: ✿ ✿ ✿
Cleanliness: ✿ ✿ ✿

KEY INFORMATION

ADDRESS:	Bradshaw Ranger District 344 South Cortez Street Prescott, AZ 86303
OPERATED BY:	Prescott National Forest
INFORMATION:	(928) 443-8000, www.fs.fed.us/r3/prescott
OPEN:	May 1–October 31
SITES:	20
EACH SITE:	Picnic table, fire ring
ASSIGNMENT:	First come, first served; reservations accepted for group site
REGISTRATION:	On-site self-registration
FACILITIES:	Vault toilets, campground host, firewood
PARKING:	At campsites
FEE:	$6
ELEVATION:	6,000 feet
RESTRICTIONS:	*Pets:* On leash only *Fires:* In fire rings only *Alcohol:* Permitted *Vehicles:* 40-foot length limit; 2 vehicles per site *Other:* 14-day stay limit; firearms prohibited; no drinking water available; 10 people per site; quiet hours 10 p.m.–6 a.m.

glimpse of a view through the ponderosas and oaks in site 15, plus a nice tent spot. Our favorite, site 16, delivers a view into a richly forested area of the creek bed and the most privacy in the campground—after a short walk from the parking tab.

The remaining sites lie on the north side of FR 97, across from the western end of the main loop. If you like the high ground, head for sites 19 and 20, uphill from the parking and overlooking the rest of the campground. Site 19 has a couple of good, well-screened tent spots. Just up the road to the east is Upper Wolf Creek, a group campground that can accommodate up to 100 people. Reservations are required and can be made online at **www.recreation.gov** or by calling (877) 444-6777.

Summer visitors from the low desert will find it pleasantly cool here, with temperatures averaging at least 20 degrees cooler than in Phoenix. Be prepared for sudden thunderstorms during the months of July through September. Lower Wolf Creek shines in fall; in September and October, the Gambel oaks and walnuts become a patchwork of gold and copper.

For a nice 8-mile loop hike through ponderosa and fir, drive north on Senator Highway to the Groom Creek Equestrian Camp. Park at the trailhead across the street from the campground. The Groom Creek Loop Trail #307 will take you past the fire lookout tower, which you can climb if manned and see all the way to the San Francisco Peaks and the Mogollon Rim. Watch your step along the path, as you'll likely share the trail with equestrians (as well as bicyclists).

If the campground is full or just too crowded for you, feel free to find your own private piece of the forest. Several designated dispersed camping sites are available along FR 74 to the west of the campground. You may also continue south down the Senator Highway to reach additional dispersed sites. A metal post that proclaims "dispersed campsite" marks each one. You'll find a fire pit, but usually no other amenities. There's no fee, of course, and you may stay in a dispersed site for 7 days in any 30-day period.

If you have the time, loop back to Prescott by going south on the Senator Highway to Walker Road. The road winds precariously through the forest, past

MAP

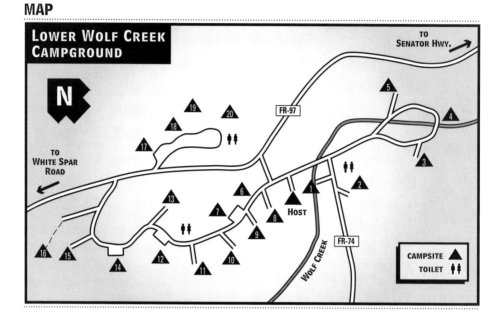

LOWER WOLF CREEK CAMPGROUND

TO SENATOR HWY.

N

FR-97

TO WHITE SPAR ROAD

HOST

WOLF CREEK

FR-74

| CAMPSITE | ▲ |
| TOILET | 👫 |

vacation homes, and eventually up to Lynx Lake. Spend the day trout fishing on this 55-acre lake, rent a kayak from the Lynx Lake Store and Marina, or stroll the paved lakeshore path and watch the cormorants hold their wings out to dry. A flash of black and white in the distance could be an osprey or a bald eagle, or closer at hand, a tiny bridled titmouse.

For a fun four-wheel-drive adventure, take Senator Highway south to Palace Station, an old stagecoach station between Phoenix and Prescott. Built in 1873, Palace Station is now listed on the National Register of Historic Places. Continue into the Bradshaw Mountains to Crown King, an old mining town turned tourist destination. For more details about the Crown King area, see profile 17, Hazlett Hollow Campground.

GETTING THERE

From Prescott, take the Senator Highway (Mt. Vernon Avenue) south 6 miles to FR 97. Turn right and drive west 1.25 miles to the campground entrance. Turn left into the campground.
Alternate route:
From Prescott, take US 89 (White Spar Road) south 6 miles to FR 97. Turn left and drive east 5.1 miles to the campground. Turn right into the campground.

GPS COORDINATES

Zone 12S
Easting 365853
Northing 3813582
North 34° 27' 18.24"
West 112° 27' 37.44"

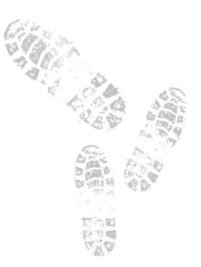

"During the spring snowmelt, the wash may be a running stream."

POWELL SPRINGS IS ONLY 15 MILES from Arizona's central corridor and Interstate 17, but it feels as if you're in the middle of nowhere. Forest Road 372 brings you up from the junction with AZ 169 through low chaparral, sometimes turning sandy as it winds through the washes below the Black Hills. The campground is at 5,300 feet elevation but is shaded by a surprising grove of ponderosa pines, along with scrub oak and alligator juniper. Wild grape vines add a touch of verdant green. The area is peppered with springs and crisscrossed with streambeds, but after years of drought, most run only after heavy rains. Powell Springs still produces clear, fresh water, but the spigot in the campground was locked down after reckless campers broke the pump twice. When the hosts are in residence, you can get a taste of spring water from the wellhead a short distance up the trail at the end of the campground. A family of harrier hawks nests annually in the canyon, and they may sweep past you as you sip, calling shrilly to one another and swooping dangerously through the trees.

Like so many of Arizona's campgrounds, Powell Springs was built by the Civilian Conservation Corps in the 1930s and has the stonework to prove it. The masonry pillar near site 11 may look like a chimney, but we're told it was once the only postal drop for the vicinity, including the nearby town of Cherry. The sites are leveled, and most are raised above the parking areas and surrounded by low stone walls. Most sites have the original fieldstone tables and sunken fire pits, with the addition of standing grills. The first three sites are well spaced under the tall pines, with morning and evening shade. We found the host conscientiously clearing the underbrush between the sites, for fire safety as well as aesthetics, so it's fairly open. Sites 4 and 8 are quite close to the camp road and have hearths instead

RATINGS

Beauty: ☆ ☆ ☆
Privacy: ☆ ☆ ☆
Spaciousness: ☆ ☆ ☆
Quiet: ☆ ☆ ☆ ☆
Security: ☆ ☆ ☆
Cleanliness: ☆ ☆ ☆ ☆

of fire pits. If you're here in the off-season, site 5 is spacious and shady, with generous parking and a large tent spot; in season this is where you'll find the host. Past the modern vault toilets, sites 6 and 7 are open and less shady. The remaining sites back up to the wash that borders the campground. During the spring snowmelt, the wash may be a running stream. Site 9 has a small tent area, but is nicely separated and lightly screened.

The campground is accessible all year, and is hosted and well maintained during the summer (unfortunately, due to the continuing budget squeeze, the Forest Service is considering leaving the campground unhosted in the future). Summer evenings cool off here, but it can be hot when the sun is up; winters are crisp to downright cold. Brief flash floods after heavy monsoon rains can cause washouts on the road, but in normal conditions a passenger car should be fine.

Leaving camp, head north on FR 372. Shortly before you reach the tiny town of Cherry, you can turn northwest on FR 132, part of the Great Western Trail. This combination route of byways, forest roads, and jeep trails runs from Mexico to Canada through some of the West's most spectacular country; this short-but-rugged section takes you toward Mingus Mountain and the fun and funky town of Jerome (for details see profile 12, Mingus Mountain Campground). Swing east at this junction and you're quickly in Cherry, which began life as a stage stop on the route between Prescott (then Fort Whipple) and Camp Verde. It's now a charming little community of summer homes with one bed-and-breakfast and some ghostly remnants of its mining-town past. No services are available.

As you leave Cherry, the road begins its descent toward the Verde River, and the red ramparts of the western Mogollon Rim are visible across the valley. Take your time on this lovely drive down to Camp Verde, where you can explore Arizona's difficult frontier years at Fort Verde State Historical Park. This was one of General George Crook's headquarters during the Apache Wars. If you'd like to go farther back in time, you're very close to Montezuma Castle National Monument, with its beautifully preserved 20-room Sinagua cliff house and Montezuma Well, a unique geological

MAP

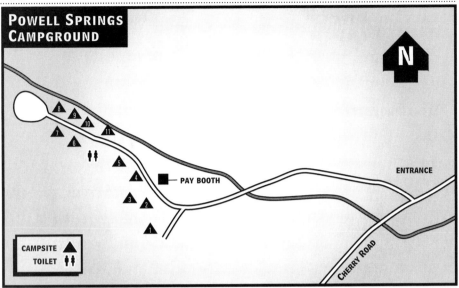

POWELL SPRINGS CAMPGROUND

N

8 9 10 11 7 6 5 4 3 2 1

PAY BOOTH

ENTRANCE

CAMPSITE
TOILET

CHERRY ROAD

GETTING THERE

From Dewey, take AZ 169 northeast 9.5 miles to FR 372 (Cherry Road). Turn left and continue north 4 miles to the campground entrance. Turn left into the campground.

oasis with life-forms found nowhere else. To spend some time enjoying the Verde, Arizona's only designated Wild and Scenic river, turn west on AZ 260 to Cottonwood and Dead Horse Ranch State Park. The Verde River Greenway, a 6-mile stretch of the river, offers a rare cottonwood-and-willow riparian forest habitat and you'll find terrific wildlife-spotting and bird-watching opportunities here. For canoeists and kayakers, there's also a paddle trail along this stretch of the river.

GPS COORDINATES

Zone 12S
Easting 402288
Northing 3826727
North 34° 34' 39.66"
West 112° 3' 55.20"

ANY PROPERTY NEAR COOL, rushing water in the arid Arizona desert is prime real estate, so it's no surprise that Beaver Creek Campground routinely fills up all year long. Thirteen sites are cradled between two arms of perennial Wet Beaver Creek, which runs clear and strong below Sedona-red bluffs. Arizona sycamores, cottonwoods, and junipers line the creek bed, shading the chuckling stream and most of the campsites.

Check in with the camp host at site 12 when you arrive. Forest Service concessionaire Recreation Resource Management hosts the campground year-round. The first four sites on the right are a little close to their neighbors, but they're also close to the creek. Each has a flat, diagonal parking tab suitable for a pop-up trailer or pickup truck, but the short vehicle length limit (22 feet) will keep the bigger RVs from moving in. Site 1 is probably the shadiest of these sites. Site 4 would make a nice choice because the tent area and fire pit are on the creek side of the site, away from the camp road. Roomy, popular sites 5 and 6 sit on level red sand where the creek curves around the campground. The song of the creek is brightest here, but there's no shade, so bring your portable canopy and sunscreen.

Compact site 7 has a secluded tent spot hidden in the brush and offers access to the point between the two arms of the stream. If you like your privacy, site 8 is back in the corner of the loop, sheltered behind its own parking. Sites 7 through 9 are separated from the creek's drier arm by a rock berm, which theoretically prevents the campground from flooding (although in recent heavy rains Mother Nature has put this to the test).

Site 10, in the loop's center, is the only site with a long parking pullout that would accommodate a large trailer. You'll have lots of room to spread out in this open area, but as you're placing your tent, plan for

> *The stream is regularly stocked with trout, and the campground is stocked with regulars.*

RATINGS

Beauty: ☆ ☆ ☆ ☆
Privacy: ☆ ☆ ☆
Spaciousness: ☆ ☆ ☆
Quiet: ☆ ☆ ☆
Security: ☆ ☆ ☆ ☆
Cleanliness: ☆ ☆ ☆ ☆ ☆

KEY INFORMATION

unthinking campers making a beeline to the toilets. Sites 11 and 13 are on either side of the host's trailer; junipers and sycamores nicely shade site 11, and site 13 has a cool tent spot a bit apart from the picnic table and fire pit.

A path running between sites 2 and 3 leads down to the creek. Wet Beaver Creek is spring fed, and its level fluctuates with the snowmelt and rain runoff from higher ground near Flagstaff. The stream is regularly stocked with trout, and the campground is stocked with regulars who return most weekends to cast a hopeful line. November is the most popular month of all, when the sycamores' broad leaves change colors.

Across the road from the campground is a no-fee area with picnic tables and upright grills (no overnight camping here). From the picnic area you can follow any of the many paths down to the creek to reach private fishing spots or cool swimming holes. Just west on Forest Road 618, turn at the historic Beaver Creek Ranger Station for the trailhead to access the Wet Beaver Creek Wilderness. The Bell Trail #13, Apache Maid Trail #15, and White Mesa Trail #86 provide 25 miles of splendid hiking in and around Wet Beaver Creek Canyon.

East on FR 618 is the V Bar V Heritage site, the largest petroglyph site in the Verde Valley. Thought to have been scribed by the Sinagua people, this mysterious aggregation of ancient signs had one use still apparent today, as a solar calendar. Two protruding rocks cast parallel shadows, creating a shaft of sunlight that spotlights particular petroglyphs marking the winter and summer solstice, and perhaps other milestones such as planting and harvest times. A $5 per vehicle fee (or a Red Rock Pass) and a short walk gets you to the petroglyphs, but leave the pooch behind since pets are not allowed. Farther down FR 618, you will come to FR 215, the turnoff for Bull Pen Dispersed Area. This primitive creekside camp is nice and shady, but in some disarray from recent flooding. Locals tell us that it's occasionally known for wildlife in the form of rowdy Camp Verde teenagers.

MAP

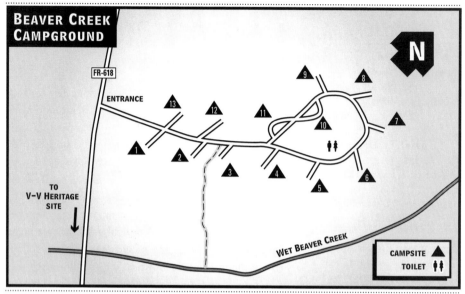

BEAVER CREEK CAMPGROUND

FR-618

ENTRANCE

TO
V-V HERITAGE
SITE

WET BEAVER CREEK

N

CAMPSITE ▲
TOILET ♂♀

From Beaver Creek it's a quick trip to Montezuma Well, a natural limestone sink that receives more than 1 million gallons of 75°F water daily from warm underground streams. Because of this the well has developed its own unique ecology; it teems with leeches, shrimp-like amphipods, water scorpions, and algae. Thousands of years ago, the Sinagua irrigated their crops by diverting the water from the Well, and it still provides water to local farmers. The eponymous Aztec emperor never set foot here, but you can learn more about the Sinagua by traveling a bit farther south and visiting the beautifully preserved cliff dwellings at Montezuma Castle National Monument.

If you need supplies, you can find almost anything in nearby Camp Verde, including the world's largest Kokopelli, a 32-foot, five-ton tribute to the flute-playing fertility figure. Many more hiking and adventuring opportunities can be found in the Sedona area, just across Interstate 17 to the west. For other area details see the Powell Springs (15) and Manzanita (10) profiles.

GETTING THERE

From Camp Verde, take I-17 north to FR 618 (exit 298). Turn right and head east 2.5 miles to the campground entrance. Turn left into the campground.

GPS COORDINATES

Zone 12S

Easting 434570

Northing 3836632

North 34° 40' 10.44"

West 111° 42' 51.00"

**THE BEST
IN TENT
CAMPING
ARIZONA**

> *See the handiwork of the Civilian Conservation Corps in the stone walls and steps leading up to restored Adirondack shelters.*

WEND YOUR WAY NORTH up Interstate 17 through the Aqua Fria River valley from Phoenix to Flagstaff, and even before you've left the saguaros behind, the rugged Bradshaw Mountains rise to the west. Tucked secretively in the forested interior is the thriving hamlet of Crown King. Named after the Crowned King mine, the town once served as the center of a bustling mining district and today is a popular tourist destination and summer retreat.

Leave the highway at the signs for the Horsethief Basin Recreation Area and pass through tiny Cleator. As you begin to climb into the hills, the road follows the route of "Murphy's Impossible Railroad." In the late 1800s, naysayers doubted entrepreneur Frank Murphy could build a railroad through these rocky mountains to the valley of Mayer. But Murphy made it happen: completed in 1904, it successfully transported more than $1 million worth of ore. The rails were taken up in 1927, but the gentle grade and narrow passages cut through walls of rock remain. At the hairpin turns look for the areas where the train was switched onto a spur, backed up the next slope, switched onto another spur, then pulled forward again; the process that gave us the word *switchback*.

Near the now-collapsed railway tunnel, you'll turn through a narrow passage (watch out for ATVs) and suddenly find yourself "downtown" amongst the trees. Turn right to check out the Crown King Saloon, heroically saved from several historic fires even as other buildings burned. During one early incident, quick-thinking miners reduced the potential flammability of the saloon by drinking its entire contents. The upstairs rooms from its bordello days are now available for legitimate lodging. Load up with homemade fudge from the General Store or have some Thrifty ice cream at the Rocky Road Sweet Stop, then continue down Forest

RATINGS

Beauty: ✩ ✩ ✩
Privacy: ✩ ✩ ✩ ✩
Spaciousness: ✩ ✩ ✩
Quiet: ✩ ✩ ✩
Security: ✩ ✩ ✩
Cleanliness: ✩ ✩

Road 52 for 7 miles to Hazlett Hollow. The road gets rougher past Crown King, and high clearance is recommended. If you prefer to camp on your own piece of mountain, you'll find several dispersed camping spots among the boulders and pines along the road.

On your way to Horsethief Basin, you climb higher into clearings affording you grand vistas across the mountains all the way to Phoenix. Outlaws based here once stole horses from Phoenix, changed their brands in the remote valley, sold them in Prescott, and then repeated the process headed in the other direction. The picturesque cabin on your right as you reach the recreation area is available for rent from the Forest Service as part of their Rooms With a View program. Just up the road opposite the cabin is Horsethief Lake, stocked with largemouth bass, sunfish, and catfish. For a nice short hike, walk across the dam and follow a footpath around the small lake.

As you pull into the campground, look for the handiwork of the Civilian Conservation Corps in the stone walls and steps leading up to restored Adirondack shelters. There are no purpose-made tent pads, but only site 15 lacks a good spot. To experience camping as it was in the 1940s, you can always set up your cot in the shelter.

Set in a small, steep valley, the scrub oak and ponderosas provide screening and shade. The sites on the outside of the loop are more private and well separated. Site 14 at the end of the loop has a nice layout with large tenting areas and a level parking tab. Sites 12 and 13 sit very close together and would accommodate two families or a group. Our favorites are sites 6, 7, and 9, with no close neighbors and shelters facing the woods. For sites without steps, choose one inside the loop, but beware of rattlesnakes down in the wash.

Technically ATVs and motorbikes are prohibited in the Horsethief Basin Recreation Area and Hazlett Hollow Campground, but they're a primary form of transportation as well as recreation in this area. Folks camping in the forest sometimes drive through the campground to use the facilities. The campground is not hosted, and it shows signs of wear and tear, but it has plenty of charm to compensate.

KEY INFORMATION

ADDRESS: Bradshaw Ranger District 344 South Cortez Street Prescott, AZ 86303

OPERATED BY: Prescott National Forest

INFORMATION: (928) 443-8000, www.fs.fed.us/r3/prescott

OPEN: May 1–October 1

SITES: 15

EACH SITE: Adirondack shelter, picnic table, fire ring, standing grill

ASSIGNMENT: First come, first served; no reservations

REGISTRATION: On-site self-registration

FACILITIES: Vault toilets, water spigots

PARKING: At campsites

FEE: $6

ELEVATION: 6,000 feet

RESTRICTIONS: *Pets:* On leash only
Fires: In fire rings only
Alcohol: Permitted
Vehicles: 32-foot length limit; No ATVs, no motorbikes, high clearance recommended
Other: 14-day stay limit; bear country food-storage restrictions; firearms prohibited; quiet hours 10 p.m.–6 a.m.; 10 people per site; checkout 2 p.m.

MAP

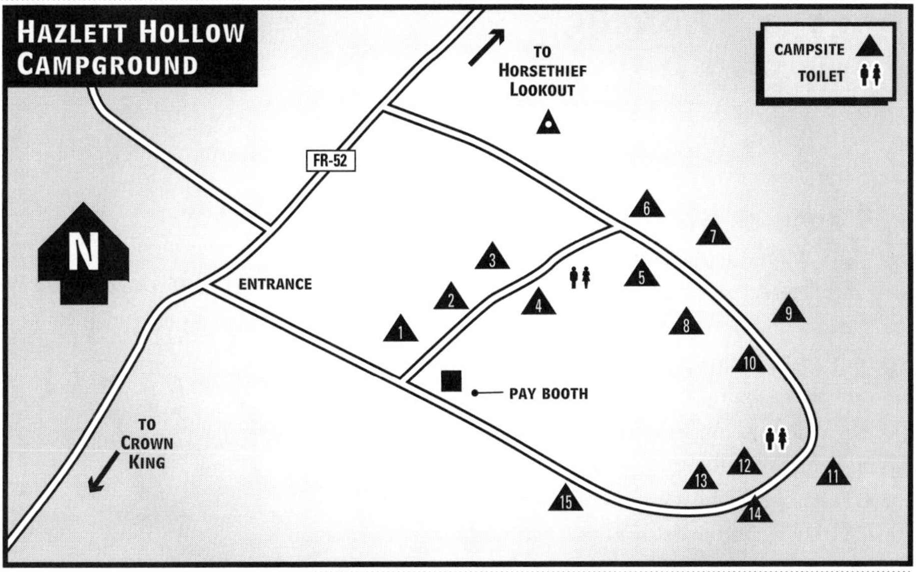

HAZLETT HOLLOW CAMPGROUND
TO HORSETHIEF LOOKOUT
CAMPSITE
TOILET
FR-52
N
ENTRANCE
PAY BOOTH
TO CROWN KING
1
2
3
4
5
6
7
8
9
10
11
12
13
14
15

GETTING THERE

From Crown King, take FR 52 southeast 7 miles to the campground.

GPS COORDINATES

Zone 12S
Easting 381358
Northing 3781793
North 34° 10' 13.26"
West 112° 17' 14.16"

A mile farther on is Kentuck Springs, a campground that's been converted to day use. Access may be restricted due to standing dead timber, and you may find prescribed burns in progress as the Forest Service tries to restore the forest's health. FR 52 climbs steeply past this point, but persevere to the historic Horsethief fire lookout tower, where on a clear day you can see all the way from Phoenix's South Mountain to Flagstaff's San Francisco Peaks. If the fireguard on duty is Tony Nelson, a pioneer son of Crown King, he can fill you in on local history.

There's a lot of great hiking around the southern Bradshaws, so check in with the Forest Service to find out more about Algonquin, Castle Creek, Horsethief Canyon, East Fort, and other trails. For a civilized touch to your experience, head back into Crown King for a gourmet surf and turf meal at the Mill Restaurant (where the centerpiece is the massive ore-crushing stamp mill from the old Gladiator Mine), then join the crowd at the Saloon for a drink and live music.

18
DESERT TORTOISE
CAMPGROUND

ARIZONANS LIKE TO BOAST that we have more boats per capita than any other state. Whether this is true or not, you'll believe it on a hot day at Lake Pleasant. If you can't escape the valley entirely when it's 100°F in the shade, the next best thing is to find the nearest large body of water. For a lot of metropolitan Phoenix, this is it. In spring and fall, and even at the height of summer, you can expect the lake to be covered in boats and the shoreline dotted with people.

Two campgrounds accommodate the many visitors to Lake Pleasant: Desert Tortoise and Roadrunner. Roadrunner's 72 developed sites sit atop the hill near the visitor center, overlooking the lake. These sites provide electricity and water and, unsurprisingly, are popular with RVs. In the three loops of Desert Tortoise, you can choose among developed, semideveloped, or tent sites. The campground sits right at the water's edge, and most sites have great views of the lake.

Pass by the Scute loop, the first turn along Desert Tortoise Road. These sites are at the tail-end of Sunset Cove, a narrow inlet that turns dry when the water level is low. Instead, turn into the Bajada loop. On the right, look for site 133, just below the road across from the restrooms. This walk-in site claims its own promontory, and the water is just a short scramble down a rocky slope. Your view from here looks down the cove to the lake, and you may feel like your tent is a tiny castle. Turn at the restroom and head uphill around the one-way loop to reach the highest part of the peninsula, where you have a bird's-eye view of the lake. As you round the loop you come to two of our favorite sites, 159 and 160. The sites are 50 and 100 feet from the parking, screened by paloverde and other desert scrub brush. If you brought along your kayak or canoe, you can portage down to the shore and begin exploring the lake right from your campsite. Water and electricity seem

> *Portage down to the shore and begin exploring the lake right from your campsite.*

RATINGS

Beauty: ✿ ✿ ✿ ✿
Privacy: ✿ ✿ ✿
Spaciousness: ✿ ✿ ✿
Quiet: ✿ ✿
Security: ✿ ✿ ✿ ✿
Cleanliness: ✿ ✿ ✿ ✿

incongruous at a walk-in tent site, but the entire loop is developed and will allow you to camp in luxury if you choose. If you have a portable evaporative cooler, it might almost make summer camping here bearable. Continuing around the loop, you will come to another parking area for two more tent sites, 161 and 162, whose main attraction is the view. If you didn't bring anything with a plug, continue down Desert Tortoise Road to the Pallet Loop. After passing the campground host's site, you'll find six sites on your left. While not well screened from each other, they're just fine if you like an open feeling and a terrific view. Below the road on your right are five more tent sites, 166 through 170. Park at the shared parking lot and climb down a few steps to reach them. The first four are all in a row, cascading down toward the water, just a short walk away. The fifth is off by itself just below the road. All sites have a small shade ramada, but be forewarned that the summer months are scorchers. On the other hand, if you've got a good sleeping bag for chilly nights, mid-winter can offer perfect days for hiking the 2-mile Pipeline Canyon Trail, with far less of a crowd in camp. You're also welcome to dry camp anywhere along the shoreline. If you continue down Desert Tortoise Road, don't speed, because the pavement goes right into the water. People who've come to scuba dive often park or camp here, making it easy to get their equipment into the water. Boating and fishing are, naturally, the primary activities on the lake. The lake hosts more than a dozen species of fish, including introduced species such as tilapia and white crappie. You'll find two boat ramps, one of them ten lanes wide, and both provide ample parking. Don't have a boat? Don't worry, the Pleasant Harbor Marina offers

KEY INFORMATION

ADDRESS: Lake Pleasant Regional Park, 41835 N. Castle Hot Springs Road, Morristown, AZ 85342

OPERATED BY: Maricopa County Parks and Recreation Department

INFORMATION: (928) 501-1710, www.maricopa.gov/parks/lake_pleasant

OPEN: Year-round

SITES: 76 (10 walk-in tent sites)

EACH SITE: Picnic table, fire ring, ramada, water spigots at some, electrical hookups at some

ASSIGNMENT: First come, first served; no reservations

REGISTRATION: Purchase daily and annual passes at the park entrance station; use self-pay station when entrance station closed

FACILITIES: Flush toilets, hot showers, water spigots, boat ramp, picnic shelters, pay phone, dump station, interpretive activities and programs, water at visitor center, drinking fountains, group sites, campground host, handicap-accessible sites, firewood

PARKING: At campsites

FEE: $10–$20

ELEVATION: 1,700 feet

RESTRICTIONS: *Pets:* On leash only. *Fires:* In fire rings only. *Alcohol:* Permitted. *Vehicles:* 50-foot length limit; 2 vehicles per site; off-road driving prohibited. *Other:* 14-day stay limit; 8 people per site; 2 tents per site; state fishing permits required; glass bottles prohibited; loaded firearms prohibited; removal of vegetation prohibited; quiet hours 10 p.m.–6 a.m.

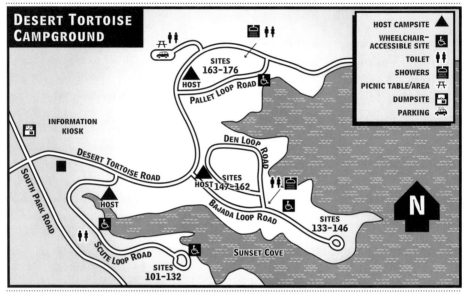

DESERT TORTOISE CAMPGROUND

SITES 163–176
HOST
PALLET LOOP ROAD
INFORMATION KIOSK
DEN LOOP ROAD
DESERT TORTOISE ROAD
HOST SITES 147–162
SOUTH PARK ROAD
HOST
BAJADA LOOP ROAD
SITES 133–146
SCUTE LOOP ROAD
SUNSET COVE
SITES 101–132

HOST CAMPSITE
WHEELCHAIR-ACCESSIBLE SITE
TOILET
SHOWERS
PICNIC TABLE/AREA
DUMPSITE
PARKING

N

boat and Jet Ski rentals. Splash through the lake on an Arizona Ducks tour in World War II–vintage amphibious vehicles. You can also purchase anything you need at The Village Store, or enjoy a meal at the Waterfront Bar and Grill. Lake Pleasant continues to improve the facilities, with a new marina being constructed at Scorpion Bay and plans for a swimming beach.

Check the events calendar online or at the visitor center for information and details about upcoming ranger-led hikes and kayak/canoe tours, children's activities, educational programs, and fishing and wakeboarding tournaments. The Desert Outdoor Center, located at the southeastern edge of the lake, is an old guest ranch that can be reserved for educational programs, weddings, and business meetings; contact them for dates for the next stargazing party or guided hiking tours open to the public. Lake Pleasant was formed by damming the Agua Fria River, which feeds into the lake from the northeast. At the visitor center you can learn more about seasonal closures of the Agua Fria inlet for nesting bald eagles, as well as see local critters, including a live Gila monster and a tarantula.

GETTING THERE

From Phoenix, take I-17 north to the Carefree Highway (AZ 74), exit 223. Turn left and drive northwest 11.2 miles to Castle Hot Springs Road. Turn right and head north 2.2 miles to Lake Pleasant Access Road. Turn right and drive 0.3 miles to the park entrance station. Continue 0.45 miles to South Park Road. Turn right and drive south 0.27 miles to Desert Tortoise Road.

GPS COORDINATES

Zone 12S
Easting 378990
Northing 3747505
North 33° 51' 39.30"
West 112° 18' 29.52"

19
THE POINT CAMGROUND

> *A great place to go to escape the city.*

AS THE SALT RIVER WINDS DOWN to the Valley of the Sun, it has carved deep and sometimes spectacular canyons. In the narrow passage between the Mazatzal and Superstition mountains, the canyon has been dammed to create four deep reservoirs that feed the mighty thirst of Phoenix. Read running upriver, their names form the mnemonic SCAR: Saguaro, Canyon, Apache, and Roosevelt. On Canyon Lake you'll find the unusual camping opportunity of three nicely developed sites with facilities—and no road access at all. Transfer your car camping gear to something that floats a little better and enjoy a night at The Point.

Before you leave, get your Tonto Pass. Canyon Lake is in Tonto National Forest, and you'll have to buy a daily recreation pass, but you can't purchase one at the lake. If you plan to camp, get enough passes to cover each day you'll be in the national forest. More information about the Tonto Pass can be found under Permits and Access in the Introduction on page 7.

Follow the historic Apache Trail as it twists and winds its way through the saguaro-studded canyon. Stop at the overlook just before you begin the final descent to get a bird's-eye view of the lake's main basin, deep-blue water patterned by white wakes. Past the final curve, look down from the one-lane bridge that spans First Water Cove to see who's fishing the quiet inlet. The lake is routinely stocked with rainbow trout and produces record-breaking largemouth bass. The creased canyon walls form many coves for fish and fishermen to explore.

If you've brought your own boat, you can launch from either the Palo Verde or Laguna boating sites. Palo Verde is probably the better choice for paddlers, as it's a bit closer to The Point. If you're boatless, Canyon Lake Marina offers rentals ranging from kayaks to

RATINGS

Beauty: ✩ ✩ ✩ ✩
Privacy: ✩ ✩ ✩
Spaciousness: ✩ ✩ ✩ ✩
Quiet: ✩ ✩
Security: ✩ ✩
Cleanliness: ✩ ✩

pontoon party barges. As you might expect this close to Phoenix, this can be a very crowded lake. On weekends from April through October, it often reaches maximum boating capacity early in the day, so arrive early or be prepared to wait for someone else to pull out.

Across the broad stretch of water from the marina, you'll see boats running at full speed seemingly disappear into the unforgiving cliffs. They're not suicidal; they're actually following the river as it winds its way to the northeast, eventually reaching Horse Mesa Dam on Apache Lake. Your destination lies up this sheer, snaking, stone corridor. The official direction of lake traffic is counterclockwise, but few seem to care, so keep your eyes peeled for distracted ski-boat drivers and Jet Ski cowboys. Canoes and kayaks will be safest sticking to the shoreline, where you're rewarded with the company of great blue herons and curious grebes, and you may even glimpse bighorn sheep on narrow canyon ledges.

Three miles up the lake, three campsites on a headland jutting from the northern shore comprise The Point Campground. The dock can easily accommodate several boats, and a short uphill trail leads to the three sites and restroom building. As the only proper bathroom on the upper part of the lake, it sees a lot of day (and some night) use. Each of the three sites has a sizable shade ramada that covers the picnic table as well as a large, flat area to pitch your tent. This was a great idea on someone's part, since the temperature difference between shade and sun can be significant any time of the year. Each site has an upright grill and a steel fire pit, so be sure to bring the barbecue supplies.

Site 1 is convenient to the dock, but could use a little more screening from the restroom foot traffic. Site 3, which sits above and behind the restroom, has plenty of privacy, yet a nice open feeling and great views. Our pick is site 2, farthest from the dock and most secluded. The ground cover is surprisingly dense with mesquite, paloverde trees, brittlebush, jojoba, and cholla, and all three sites are strategically placed so that you can't see your neighbors. In spring, blooming brittlebush envelope the sites in yellow, with orange globemallow and purple scorpionweed adding extra color.

KEY INFORMATION

ADDRESS:	Mesa Ranger Station 5140 East Ingram Street Mesa, AZ 85205
OPERATED BY:	Tonto National Forest
INFORMATION:	(480) 610-3300, www.fs.fed.us/r3/tonto
OPEN:	Year-round
SITES:	3
EACH SITE:	Picnic table, fire ring, upright grill, ramada
ASSIGNMENT:	First come, first served; no reservations
REGISTRATION:	None required; purchase daily Tonto Pass before arriving
FACILITIES:	Composting toilets, boat dock, emergency phone
PARKING:	At Palo Verde Boating Site, Canyon Lake Marina, or Laguna Boating Site
FEE:	$6 per vehicle; $4 per watercraft
ELEVATION:	1,700 feet
RESTRICTIONS:	*Pets:* On leash only *Fires:* In fire rings *Alcohol:* Permitted *Vehicles:* Access by boat only *Other:* 14-day stay limit; pack-in/out; discharging firearms prohibited; no drinking water; horses, glass containers prohibited; soaps/detergents prohibited in lake; quiet hours 10 p.m.–6 a.m.

MAP

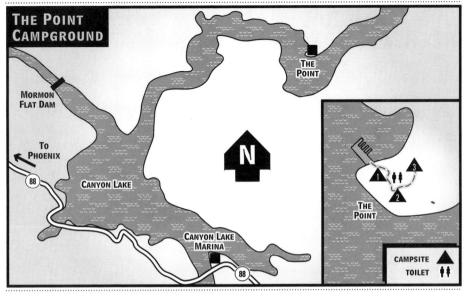

THE POINT CAMPGROUND

MORMON FLAT DAM

TO PHOENIX

88

CANYON LAKE

THE POINT

CANYON LAKE MARINA

88

THE POINT

1   2   3

CAMPSITE ▲
TOILET ♀♂

GETTING THERE

From Phoenix, take US 60 east to Idaho Road, exit 196. Turn left and go north 2.25 miles to AZ 88. Turn right and head northeast 13.5 miles to the lake.

GPS COORDINATES

Zone 12S

Easting 461804

Northing 2713161

North 33° 33' 26.70"

West 111° 24' 41.34"

The Point Campground is a great place to escape the city, indulge in cool, splashy fun, and spend a night under the stars, but we won't fib to you: there's not a lot of peace or solitude here. The canyon walls amplify the growl of engines day and night, and you won't spend much time out of sight of other people. If you get the chance, come midweek or in the off-season.

The Maricopa County Sheriff's Office, Arizona Game and Fish, and the Forest Service all police the lake. An emergency call box on the restroom building should bring help if you require it. There's no drinking water and the campground is pack in/pack out, so plan accordingly. Some basic supplies, such as firewood, are available at Canyon Lake Marina, and you can always treat yourself to a meal at the cantina that overlooks the water. Next door is the berth of the *Dolly* steamboat, which chugs on leisurely, narrated cruises around the lake. Check out the Lost Dutchman (22), Burnt Corral (20), and Cholla (21) profiles for more about the canyon lakes and the Apache Trail.

20
BURNT CORRAL
RECREATION SITE

APACHE LAKE, FORMED BY HORSE MESA DAM, is the second-largest of the four reservoirs on the Salt River northeast of Phoenix. All of the lakes in the chain are more or less within easy reach of the Phoenix metropolitan area. To get to them, you twist and wind your way along the Apache Trail National Scenic Byway, past Lost Dutchman State Park and along Canyon Lake. If you've got the munchies, stop at the restaurant and general store at the ghost town of Tortilla Flat, just past Canyon Lake. The Apache Trail turns to dirt shortly after this, but is well maintained and poses no trouble for a carefully driven sedan. You might want to park at the Fish Creek bridge and hike along the canyon bottom, scrambling your own way around the boulders. After a wet season, you'll see numerous waterfalls and pools, and may even find yourself taking a compulsory swim or two. During fall or early winter, the sycamores and cottonwoods that line the creek burst into color. This area is prone to flash floods, so be sure to check the weather forecast before exploring the canyon.

Toward the eastern end of 17-mile Apache Lake, you will come to Burnt Corral Recreation Site. The campground is laid out in a long, one-way loop with bisecting roads and a couple of extra loops at the beginning and end. A host lives here in fall and winter, and bird-watchers will want to get up early to check out the crowd at the host's feeders. Sites are designated as single, double, triple, or quadruple, with corresponding limits on occupancy, but you pay the same price no matter the size of the site. Take a right up toward sites 4 through 13 if you'd like to be away from the crowds yet overlook the lake; expect these sites to be warmer, in summer or winter, than those along the shore. Creosote, jojoba, paloverde, and ocotillo surround and screen these sites. Continuing down the loop, desert

> *Burnt Corral offers plenty of shade and an unobstructed view of the lake.*

RATINGS

Beauty: ✪ ✪ ✪ ✪
Privacy: ✪ ✪ ✪
Spaciousness: ✪ ✪ ✪
Quiet: ✪ ✪
Security: ✪ ✪ ✪
Cleanliness: ✪ ✪ ✪

KEY INFORMATION

ADDRESS: Tonto Basin Ranger District HC02 P.O. Box 4800 Roosevelt, AZ 85545

OPERATED BY: Tonto National Forest

INFORMATION: (928) 467-3200, www.fs.fed.us/r3/tonto

OPEN: Year-round

SITES: 79

EACH SITE: Picnic table, fire ring, some have an upright grill, some have ramadas

ASSIGNMENT: First come, first served; no reservations

REGISTRATION: None required; purchase daily Tonto Pass before arriving

FACILITIES: Vault toilets, water spigots, boat ramp, beach, picnic area, pay phone, campground host, fish-cleaning station

PARKING: At campsites

FEE: $6 per vehicle; $4 per watercraft

ELEVATION: 1,900 feet

RESTRICTIONS: *Pets:* On leash only *Fires:* In fire rings only *Alcohol:* Permitted *Vehicles:* 22-foot length limit; 2 vehicles per site *Other:* 14-day stay limit; shooting of firearms prohibited; 10 people per site; quiet hours 8:30 p.m.–6 a.m.

vegetation gives way to a canopy of mesquite trees. The sites that don't have mesquites to shade them have thoughtfully been built with ramadas. Beware of some of the inner sites such as 15 and 25—they appear to be private, but once you set up camp you'll realize you're closer to the neighbors than you thought.

As you come around the loop, you'll see that all of the sites on the southern edge sit directly on the water. If possible, try to snag site 36, at the end of a point with a 180-degree view of the lake. Along the rocky shoreline, either mesquites or ramadas shade compact sites 37, 40, and 42. Site 44 is also on the shore, but note that it sits across from group site 31, which can accommodate several large groups. Sites 52 and 53 are across the road from the swimming beach, with plenty of shade and an unobstructed view of the lake. Screening is minimal along the lakeshore, but sites 58, 60, and 62 have a lot of space and are shaded by mature mesquites. If the campground is full or if you want a more private (and cheaper) experience, pitch your tent in the dispersed area, southeast of the campground at the mouth of a sandy wash. These more-primitive sites also have mesquite shade, picnic tables, fire rings, and nearby porta-pots.

You'll enjoy the experience more if you adjust your expectations to include plenty of other people. These lakes are always busy, especially during the hot months when Phoenicians try to escape the heat-trapping concrete city. The campground is surrounded by National Forest land, including the Four Peaks Wilderness, Three Bar Wildlife Area, and the Superstition Wilderness. Hunters camp here during the fall and winter seasons, and the area attracts serious fishermen with crappie, catfish, smallmouth bass, largemouth bass, carp, walleye, and rainbow trout. The boat ramp near the day-use picnic area has a nifty composting fish-cleaning station. A trail leaves the campground at the northern end and heads toward a great shoreline fishing spot.

When planning your visit, check **www.srpwater.com/dwr** for information on current lake levels, which can vary quite a bit. Nearby Apache Lake Marina and Resort offers boat rentals, a motel, a restaurant, and a small grocery store. Heading north, you can get close

MAP

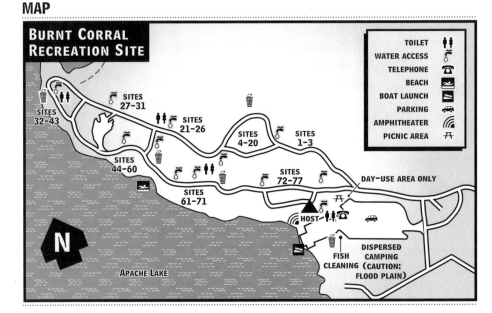

From Phoenix, take AZ 88 (the Apache Trail) north 38 miles to Forest Road 183. Turn left to the campground entrance.

to history in the Salado cliff dwellings of Tonto National Monument; see profile 21, Cholla Recreation Site, for more details.

Before you arrive, be sure to purchase your Tonto Pass. Apache Lake is in the Tonto National Forest, and you'll have to buy a daily recreation pass, but you can't purchase one at the lake. If you plan to camp, get enough passes to cover each day you'll be in the national forest. More information about the Tonto Pass can be found under Permits and Access in the Introduction on page 7.

Zone 12S

Easting 481819

Northing 3720449

North 33° 37' 25.26"

West 111° 11' 43.13"

> *If you are willing to haul your gear, you have a good chance of having prime real estate all to yourself.*

MOST PHOENICIANS KNOW SRP as the folks who send the electric bill every month, but in the early 1900s local settlers didn't worry about such newfangled stuff. They started the Salt River Project, using their land as collateral for a government loan, to build a much-needed water delivery system for their homes and crops. The loan was the first one granted under the auspices of the new National Reclamation Act in 1903, and both the dam and lake it created were named in honor of the U.S. president who helped make it possible, Theodore Roosevelt. Within a short time, turbines were installed and additional dams were built along the Salt River, including Horse Mesa Dam (which created Apache Lake), Mormon Flat Dam (Canyon Lake), and Stuart Mountain Dam (Saguaro Lake). Almost as a side effect, the area became a mecca for boaters and fishermen.

This is still a desert, however, and the U.S. Forest Service took that into account when naming Roosevelt Lake's nicest campground (also the largest all-solar-powered campground in the United States). All six loops are named after different types of cholla (pronounced choy-ah), a type of cactus with very sharp, barbed spines. The most notorious varieties are the teddy bear, which looks so soft that you are tempted to pet one (don't try it!) and the jumping cholla, which they *say* doesn't actually jump, but is devilishly clever at using your skin, clothing, or dog as transportation for propagation. Once it catches on, it's extremely reluctant to let go.

Like almost all of Arizona's lake campgrounds, Cholla was built to be RV-friendly. You could easily imagine making a home here, with hot showers, a playground for the kids, and a gorgeous view, and indeed some people now do just that. Cholla Recreation Site offers long-term stays (up to six months) between

RATINGS

Beauty: ✿ ✿ ✿ ✿
Privacy: ✿ ✿ ✿ ✿
Spaciousness: ✿ ✿ ✿
Quiet: ✿ ✿
Security: ✿ ✿ ✿ ✿
Cleanliness: ✿ ✿ ✿ ✿

October 1 and March 31, which especially appeal to snowbirds, our seasonal visitors from the snowy states. Don't despair at the sight of all the satellite dishes. You'll find 18 walk-in, tent-only sites to get away from the generators, although you can expect to hear boat engines throughout the day.

Roosevelt Lake is in the Tonto National Forest, and you'll have to buy a daily Tonto Pass before arriving since you can't purchase one at the lake. If you plan to camp, purchase one pass for each day you'll be in the national forest. More information about the Tonto Pass can be found under Permits and Access in the Introduction on page 7.

Stop at the Cane Cholla loop first. The host here says that the tent-only sites rarely get used, so if you are willing to haul your gear 50 to 400 feet from your car, you may well claim prime real estate all to yourself. Of the five sites at Cane Cholla, site 18 is the best. As the farthest site on the end of the point, it boasts terrific views up and across the lake. Jojoba, paloverde, desert broom, and Mormon tea screen the loop's sites well. Park in front of the restrooms for all five sites.

To get to the second tenting area, with 13 sites and six parking areas, continue to the last loop, Christmas Cholla. Sites 1 and 2 are adjacent, with large tent areas, and would suit a large group. The sites share great views of the Sierra Anchas and of Four Peaks. Site 3 claims the same views but is more secluded. Sites 4 and 5 sit closest to the parking area and are within sight of each other. You'll have to walk farther to sites 6 and 7, but great lake views will reward you. You can hike down to a fishing spot from the parking near site 7. Sites 8 and 9 are a good 100 feet away from the parking area and feel secluded. They look down toward Bermuda Flat, a winter migration areas for hundreds of Canada geese. Tall mesquite shrubs somewhat obscure the lake view at sites 11 through 13, but you can still enjoy the surrounding mountains. A path runs along the

KEY INFORMATION

ADDRESS:	Tonto Basin Ranger District, HC02 P.O. Box 4800, Roosevelt, AZ 85545
OPERATED BY:	Tonto National Forest
INFORMATION:	(928) 467-3200, www.fs.fed.us/r3/tonto
OPEN:	Year-round
SITES:	206
EACH SITE:	Picnic table, fire ring, ramadas
ASSIGNMENT:	First come, first served; no reservations
REGISTRATION:	None required; purchase Tonto Pass before arriving
FACILITIES:	Vault toilets, flush toilets, hot showers, water spigots, boat ramp, drinking fountains, campground host, recycling, fish-cleaning stations, fishing docks, playground
PARKING:	At campsites
FEE:	$6; $4 watercraft
ELEVATION:	2,200 feet
RESTRICTIONS:	*Pets:* On leash only. *Fires:* In fire rings only. *Alcohol:* Permitted. *Vehicles:* 32-foot length limit; 2 vehicles/1 watercraft per single site; 4 vehicles/2 watercraft per double site. *Other:* 14-day stay limit April–September; 6-month stay limit October–March; shooting of firearms prohibited; 10 people per single site; 20 people per double site

MAP

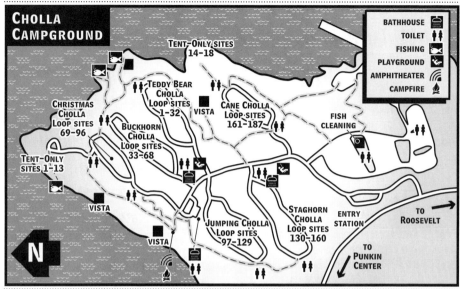

CHOLLA CAMPGROUND

BATHHOUSE
TOILET
FISHING
PLAYGROUND
AMPHITHEATER
CAMPFIRE

TENT-ONLY SITES 14-18

TEDDY BEAR CHOLLA LOOP SITES 1-32

CHRISTMAS CHOLLA LOOP SITES 69-96

VISTA

CANE CHOLLA LOOP SITES 161-187

BUCKHORN CHOLLA LOOP SITES 33-68

FISH CLEANING

TENT-ONLY SITES 1-13

VISTA

VISTA

JUMPING CHOLLA LOOP SITES 97-129

STAGHORN CHOLLA LOOP SITES 130-160

ENTRY STATION

TO ROOSEVELT

TO PUNKIN CENTER

N

GETTING THERE

From Phoenix, take AZ 87 north 60 miles to AZ 188. Turn right and drive south 28 miles to the campground.

GPS COORDINATES

Zone 12S
Easting 481009
Northing 3731509
North 33° 43' 24.30"
West 111° 12' 17.94"

outside of all the loops, connecting them and leading out to scenic overlooks. Water attracts wildlife, including geese, ducks, eagles, bighorn sheep, mule, deer, javelina, and quail. Fishermen can cast for largemouth and smallmouth bass, crappie, sunfish, catfish, and carp. Just east of the dam, Roosevelt Lake Marina offers bait and tackle, boat rentals, and lodging.

Temperatures here can easily reach a scalding 120°F in the summer, but winter days are very pleasant. Each loop has its own host, all of whom reside in the campground from November 1 to April 1. Loops close when the campground reaches capacity, with the busiest times being holiday weekends (except Christmas).

While in the area, be sure to visit Tonto National Monument and see the 700-year-old cliff dwellings of the Salado people. From the visitor center, you can climb 350 feet on the 1-mile round-trip hike to the Lower Cliff Dwelling. You must make reservations for the ranger-led tours of the Upper Cliff Dwelling, reached by climbing 600 feet in 1.5 miles. Tours are only offered November through April, and pets are not allowed on the trails.

L EGEND HAS IT THAT JACOB "THE DUTCHMAN" WALTZ FOUND GOLD while prospecting in the rugged Superstition Mountains. On his deathbed he revealed the location of his mine to two close friends, but they were unable to find it. Thousands have since gone into these mountains in search of their fortunes, and some have died trying; the Dutchman's treasure remains hidden today, even though maps to the possible location are on display at the Superstition Mountain Museum in Apache Junction. There may be no more truth to the tale than to Waltz's nickname (he was actually German), but I remember coming to the Supes for the first time as a teenager convinced I was the one who would find the lost gold. Instead I discovered an abiding love for the desert.

No trip to Phoenix is complete without a visit to the Lost Dutchman State Park. The campground makes a good fall-to-spring base camp for exploring the multiple hiking and horseback riding trails that meander through the Superstition Mountain Wilderness, 160,000 acres stretching east of Phoenix and south of the historic Apache Trail. Each campsite has a postcard-perfect backdrop of these magnificent red saguaro-studded crags.

When you first pull into the park, be sure to stop inside the visitor center to learn more about the area. If you're interested in bird-watching, pick up a birding list and point your binoculars toward the small pool along the native plant trail. Among the sparrows you may catch a glimpse of a curve-billed thrasher, a roadrunner, or a gaggle of Gambel's quail. Walk the short trail to learn the names of the plants that thrive in this desert.

Continuing into the park, a left turn takes you to the day-use areas, a right turn to the campground. Skip the first loop; you'll find sites with better screening, more privacy, and a nicer spot to pitch your tent just ahead. Heading down the road, take the second left to

> *Each campsite has a postcard-perfect backdrop of magnificent red saguaro-studded crags.*

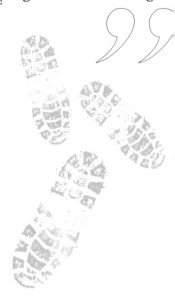

RATINGS

Beauty: ✩ ✩ ✩ ✩
Privacy: ✩ ✩ ✩
Spaciousness: ✩ ✩ ✩
Quiet: ✩ ✩ ✩
Security: ✩ ✩ ✩ ✩
Cleanliness: ✩ ✩ ✩ ✩ ✩

enter the 1 through 15 loop. These first few sites are our favorites since mature paloverde trees shade them. Because this loop only has pull-in tab parking, you are less likely to have a big RV next door. If you end up on a pull-through loop, check out sites 59 through 70, which are separated by thick brush.

If you really want privacy, you can also stay at the lone hiker/biker campsite, located along the Discovery Interpretive Trail. It's a walk of about 200 yards from parking by the showers to the site. You're also near the Siphon Draw trailhead, making this is a perfect site for an early start to your own hike. It even comes with its own bird feeder and bath.

You could hike in the Superstitions every weekend for years and never see it all. This is lowland Sonoran desert, with its signature saguaro and cholla cactus, but you'll also find tree-shaded streams and deep-canyon swimming holes hidden in these hills. From the campground, you can hike the 4-mile round-trip straight up to the towering cliffs that backdrop the campsites and into Siphon Draw Canyon. The last part of the hike up to the summit at the Flatiron is a difficult climb, 2,800 feet up on a nonmaintained trail that adds 2 miles to your hike. Just north of the state park is the easy 3-mile Massacre Grounds Trail. The trail leads you through a surreal cholla forest to the scene of a brutal 1848 confrontation between Mexican prospectors and Apaches.

Summer temperatures regularly reach the triple digits, so plan your trip for cooler weather. Winter days average in the 60s, but the sun is still intense, so wear your hat and sunscreen. Be sure to bring plenty of water with you in any season, and if you decide to try for that fabled gold, remember that treasure hunting requires a permit issued through the Tonto National Forest.

KEY INFORMATION

ADDRESS: 6109 North Apache Trail, Apache Junction, AZ 85219

OPERATED BY: Arizona State Parks

INFORMATION: (480) 982-4485, www.azstateparks.com

OPEN: Year-round

SITES: 71

EACH SITE: Picnic table, upright grill

ASSIGNMENT: First come, first served; no reservations; reservations accepted for group sites

REGISTRATION: Purchase daily and annual passes at the park office; on-site self-registration after hours

FACILITIES: Portable toilets, flush toilets, hot showers, water spigots, picnic shelters, day-use ramadas, nature trails, pay phone, dump station, amphitheater, interpretive activities and programs, guided hikes, interpretive center, drinking fountains, group sites, campground host, resident park manager, recycling

PARKING: At campsites

FEE: $12; $25 group site; $5 day use

ELEVATION: 2,000 feet

RESTRICTIONS: *Pets:* On leash only. *Fires:* No ground fires. *Alcohol:* Permitted. *Vehicles:* No length limit; 2 vehicles per site; motorized vehicles and bicycles prohibited in the Superstition Wilderness. *Other:* 15-day stay limit; firearms prohibited; firewood gathering prohibited; 12 people per site; 15-person group size in the wilderness; generator hours 8 a.m. to 9 p.m.

MAP

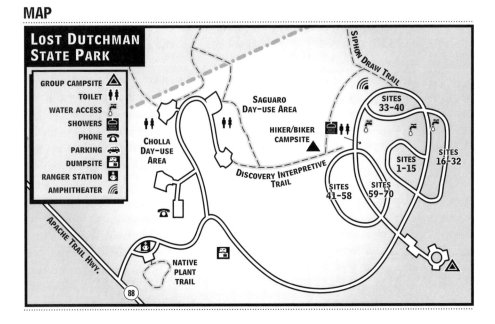

LOST DUTCHMAN STATE PARK

GROUP CAMPSITE
TOILET
WATER ACCESS
SHOWERS
PHONE
PARKING
DUMPSITE
RANGER STATION
AMPHITHEATER

CHOLLA DAY-USE AREA

SAGUARO DAY-USE AREA

HIKER/BIKER CAMPSITE

DISCOVERY INTERPRETIVE TRAIL

SIPHON DRAW TRAIL

SITES 33–40
SITES 1–15
SITES 16–32
SITES 41–58
SITES 59–70

Apache Trail Hwy.

NATIVE PLANT TRAIL

88

The Superstitions are also popular with rock climbers, especially at Weaver's Needle. This unique rock formation, created by long-ago volcanic activity, rises 4,550 feet in elevation and can be summated by experienced technical climbers. For a spectacular camping experience, haul your tent to the top of the Needle and spend the night on top of the world. Weaver's Needle can be seen from many vantage points in the Superstitions and is accessed by the Peralta Trail, off of US 60 east of Apache Junction.

Just outside the park, you can tour the old mines of Goldfield, a very productive gold mining region that some have suggested was the actual location of the Lost Dutchman Mine. Continue on AZ 88 to drive the Historic Apache Trail past Canyon Lake to the ghost town of Tortilla Flat, population six. You can saddle up at the bar in the Superstition Saloon on the saddle barstools and add your dollar bill to the wallpaper of greenbacks posted by tourists. Be sure to try the prickly pear ice cream, a sweet concoction that might sweeten your feelings toward cactus.

GETTING THERE

From Phoenix, take US 60 east to AZ 88. Turn left and head north 5 miles to the park entrance.

GPS COORDINATES

Zone 12S

Easting 455208

Northing 3702874

North 33° 27' 51.78"

West 111° 28' 55.32"

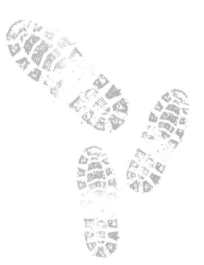

> *You won't see your neighbors from any of the sites.*

ONLY 10 MILES OF SMOOTH GRAVEL ROADS separate Pinal Peak Recreation Area from the mining meccas of Globe and Miami, but the atmosphere is a world apart. At 7,500 feet, the trees are tall and the air fresh. It's delightfully cooler than in the desert below, which persuaded many early miners to make the trek to homes up here after hard, hot workdays in the mines. Signal Peak (7,812 feet) was used by the U.S. Army as a heliograph station, allowing frontier commanders to communicate for miles by reflecting sunlight off of mirrors. Today the peaks are topped with a multitude of modern radio towers, passing messages at speeds unimaginable 150 years ago, and the heavy forest also shelters two dozen summer cabins and four campgrounds. The road is challengingly narrow, with some tight turns and great views, unobstructed by any guardrails, over the sheer slopes of the mountains.

As you enter the pines on your way up Forest Road 651, you pass the campground at Sulphide Del Rey. It's a pretty spot below the most nerve-racking parts of the road, but the campgrounds are more tent-friendly farther up the mountain. Continue to Pinal and Upper Pinal, nestled among white fir, ponderosa, and aspen near the top of the peaks. Upper Pinal, past the collection of summer cabins, consists of only three sites in a small cul-de-sac with a vault toilet, but two of the three are the shadiest, most private sites on the peak. The sites, though unnumbered, are easily recognizable, with picnic tables, fire rings, and stonework done by the Civilian Conservation Corps. The first site on the loop is uphill among the trees, invisible from the road. You'll have room to park your vehicle below the campsite but not to turn around, so you will have to back in or back out. A CCC-built wall supports a leveled site with a picnic table, a fire ring with grill, and a flat, clear

RATINGS

Beauty: ✿ ✿ ✿ ✿
Privacy: ✿ ✿ ✿ ✿
Spaciousness: ✿ ✿ ✿
Quiet: ✿ ✿ ✿ ✿
Security: ✿ ✿ ✿
Cleanliness: ✿ ✿ ✿

tent area. A trail behind you leads up toward Signal Peak and its fire tower. The table, fire ring, and standing grill at site 2 are right off of the turnaround, making this site more accommodating for those with limited mobility. A clearing big enough to set up a large tent is tucked back in the trees. Site 3, at the end of the cul-de-sac, also has a short, steep drive leading up to it. The nicely arranged site is defined by large boulders. You won't see your neighbors from any of the sites.

The campgrounds are never very crowded, but if Upper Pinal is full, you can return to Pinal and have your choice of 13 spots spread out on both sides of the road. The best sites are on the west side, on the hill at the north end of the campground. You're in alligator juniper and Gambel oak, and although your spot may have a little slope, the view from your tent across the valley below is spectacular.

You can choose among several hiking trails in these mountains, including the strenuous Sixshooter Trail #197 that leads from Icehouse CCC picnic area to the Upper Pinal campground. This 6-mile one-way hike gains 3,000 feet in elevation and passes the remains of a former sawmill and an old mine entrance. (Rumor has it that Sixshooter was so named because the sawmill workers seemed to always be packing.) You can also make a loop hike by returning on the Telephone Trail #192, which runs along an underground telephone line and provides spectacular views of Globe and Miami below. In October the mountaintop blazes as the Gambel oak, aspens, maples, velvet ash, and Arizona walnut trees change color.

Pinal Peak is known as a prolific bird-watching area, a moist sky island on the north/south divide that attracts numerous migrant species. The Peak fire in 2000 damaged the habitat and discouraged the bird-watchers, but the slow process of recovery is well on its way, and most of the birds are back. Bring your telescope as well as your spotting scope since the stars are magnificent in the dark night. Black bears and mountain lions roam here, as do whitetail and mule deer. Leave the dog dish out and you may come face-to-face with a nosy skunk (we did).

KEY INFORMATION

ADDRESS: Globe Ranger District 7680 S. Sixshooter Canyon Rd. Globe, AZ 85501

OPERATED BY: Tonto National Forest

INFORMATION: (928) 402-6200, www.fs.fed.us/r3/tonto

OPEN: May–November

SITES: 3

EACH SITE: Picnic table, fire ring, some have standing grill

ASSIGNMENT: First come, first served; no reservations

REGISTRATION: None required

FACILITIES: Vault toilets

PARKING: At campsites

FEE: Free

ELEVATION: 7,500 feet

RESTRICTIONS: *Pets:* On leash only
Fires: In fire rings only
Alcohol: Permitted
Vehicles: 16-foot length limit; no ATVs
Other: 14-day stay limit; bear country food-storage restrictions; pack in/pack out; firearms prohibited; no drinking water available

MAP

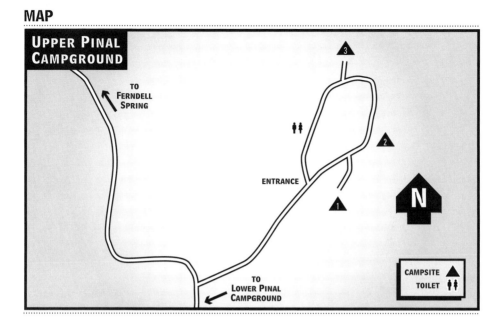

GETTING THERE

From Globe, take Jess Hayes Road southeast 2 miles to FR 112. Turn right and head south 2.5 miles to FR 55. Turn right and go southwest 2.5 miles to FR 651. Turn left and continue 10 miles to the Pinal Mountain Recreation Area. Continue 1 mile up the mountain to Upper Pinal.

GPS COORDINATES

Zone 12S
Easting 516638
Northing 3682836
North 33° 17' 04.02"
West 110° 49' 16.74"

On the other side of the mountain is Pioneer Pass Campground. This is also a lovely area, with several sites tucked behind boulders and invisible from the road. It was also developed by the CCC, and several of the original fieldstone tables and hearths can still be seen. The Kellner picnic site, which is available for large groups, is the only facility in the Pinal Mountain Recreation Area that charges a fee. Because of the lower elevation, you won't find pines, but a small stream running through the area provides sustenance for sycamores and oaks.

If you want to venture out of the campground, Globe's historic downtown displays a lot of interesting architecture from the early 1900s, and you'll find some neat antiques shops as well as many reminders of the region's ongoing mining heritage. Be sure to stop at the Besh-Ba-Gowah Archaeological Park to stand on the plaza of a partially restored 700-year-old Salado Indian pueblo, and explore the small but very informative museum.

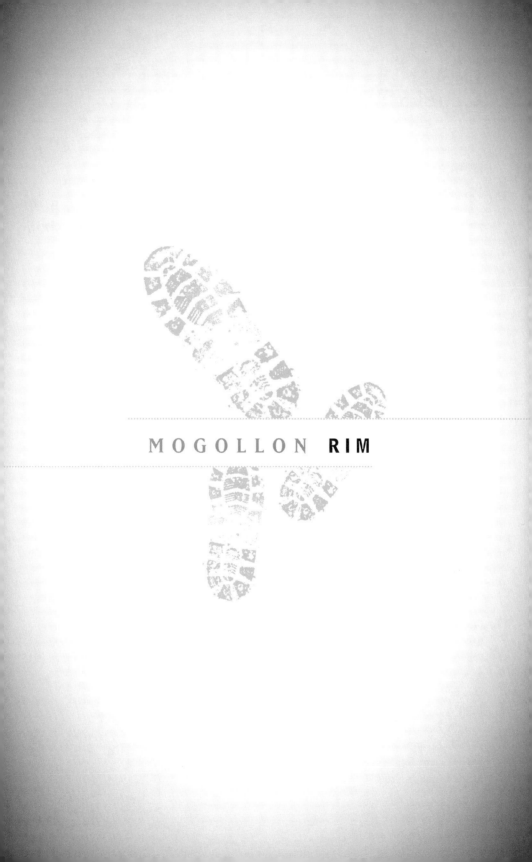

MOGOLLON **RIM**

24
CHEVELON CROSSING CAMPGROUND

THE MOGOLLON RIM AREA is known for its tall pines and crystalline, trout-stocked lakes. The General Crook National Recreation Trail and its parallel route, Forest Road 300 or the Rim Road, wend their way along the 2,000-foot escarpment from east to west. The majority of rim-country traffic stays within a few miles of this road and the well-known lakes. North of the Mogollon Rim on FR 504 is Chevelon Crossing Campground, one of the smallest and least-used of the rim campgrounds. With six sites on sloping, rocky ground in a canyon, this campground might seem an unlikely candidate for a best rating, but it's got a few outstanding features. Not the least of these is relatively light use at even the most popular times of year.

Chevelon Crossing is approachable from the south on either FR 504 or FR 169, which intersect near the bridge over Chevelon Creek. As you climb away from the rim, tall ponderosas fade into juniper and creosote, and you may wonder where you're headed, but in the canyon you find the pines again. Because the elevation is lower here than in the majority of the rim country, expect shrubbier trees and warmer summer temperatures. The campground, originally built by the Civilian Conservation Corps in the 1930s, is set on the slope of Chevelon Canyon overlooking the creek. Both are named for a trapper who died in the canyon after eating the roots of the water hemlock plant, a poisonous relative of the carrot. Steep, rock walls rise across from the campground, forming a backdrop for the trees. The rocky stream is perennial but dries up in some parts (in fact, before Chevelon had his fatal dinner, it was called Big Dry Wash), but after heavy rains large, cool swimming holes await only a mile upstream.

The campsites are best suited for smaller tents and self-sufficient campers. Each site has a good, steel picnic table and fire ring (be sure to check fire restrictions

> *Only a mile upstream large, cool swimming holes await.*

RATINGS

Beauty: ✿ ✿ ✿ ✿
Privacy: ✿ ✿ ✿
Spaciousness: ✿ ✿
Quiet: ✿ ✿ ✿
Security: ✿ ✿
Cleanliness: ✿ ✿ ✿

ADDRESS:	Black Mesa Ranger District P.O. Box 968 Overgaard, AZ 85933
OPERATED BY:	Apache-Sitgreaves National Forests
INFORMATION:	(928) 535-4481, www.fs.fed.us/r3/asnf
OPEN:	Year-round
SITES:	6
EACH SITE:	Picnic table, fire ring
ASSIGNMENT:	First come, first served; no reservations
REGISTRATION:	None required
FACILITIES:	Vault toilets
PARKING:	At campsites
FEE:	Free
ELEVATION:	6,300 feet
RESTRICTIONS:	*Pets:* On leash only *Fires:* In fire rings only *Alcohol:* Permitted *Vehicles:* 16-foot length limit *Other:* 14-day stay limit; pack in/pack out; no drinking water available

on the information board) and some privacy from the other sites. Each site also has at least a two-man tent-able area, but they're not purpose-made tent pads and may be a little sloped or rocky. There are vault toilets, but no water and no garbage service. The six unnumbered sites are arranged on the hillside in tiers, all with views across the canyon. The first three sites you come to are lined up along the creek side of the campground slightly below the road. Softer, shadier tent spots await below these sites near the creek. The third site may be the pick of the litter, with its own parking loop, shade from a big pine tree, and close proximity to the main trail that leads down to the creek. The remaining three sites are up the slope, nestled among the junipers. The fifth is nicely screened but very close to the road.

While you're at Chevelon Crossing, take time to hike along Chevelon Creek. If you're self-contained and willing to haul your gear a little way, you'll find more camping options in a meadow just a short hike up the creek (south). Be aware of your impact here and properly dispose of your solid waste. The canyon is known for a healthy population of rattlesnakes and fire ants, so keep your eyes open as you're setting up camp. The trail runs from the meadow all the way to Chevelon Lake Dam. After 2 miles the trail becomes challenging and unmaintained, but in that short distance you can find some great swimming holes and spot wildlife, including beavers, skunks, mule deer, and plenty of birds.

You can fish for brown and rainbow trout in the pools of Chevelon Creek, but if you've come to the rim for fishing, you may want to try Chevelon Lake, 11 miles south of Chevelon Crossing off of FR 169 and 169B. Chevelon Lake, with its 200 acres of surface area, is the least-accessible, most-remote lake on the rim. Near the lake is a six-site campground with vault toilets that sees a bit more use than Chevelon Crossing. On maps, FR 169B appears to continue to the lake, but in reality it becomes an extremely rocky four-wheel-drive road and is closed to anything larger than an ATV just 0.25 miles past the campground. Boats with electric or 10-horsepower gas motors or less are allowed on the lake, but have to be trekked down and back up the steep, 0.75-mile road (and boats left at the lake more

MAP

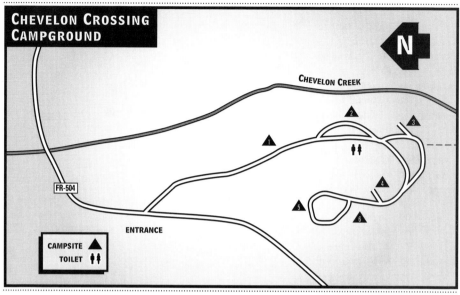

CHEVELON CROSSING CAMPGROUND

CHEVELON CREEK

N

FR-504

ENTRANCE

CAMPSITE ▲
TOILET

than 24 hours may be confiscated!) so float tubes are more popular. The difficult access is to the trout's benefit, and you may land a prizewinner here.

The trailhead sign you see in the Chevelon Crossing parking lot is not for a hiking trail—it's for the north end of the Long Draw OHV trail, which encompasses a 30-mile loop of forest roads. The south trailhead is at Chevelon Lake Campground. In either campground you may encounter ATV and dirt-bike enthusiasts, and we've seen unmistakable evidence of equestrian occupation as well, but the area is usually so quiet it's well worth taking a chance.

GETTING THERE

From Heber, take AZ 260 west 1 mile to FR 504. Turn right and drive north 18 miles to the campground.

From Winslow, take AZ 99 south 27 miles to FR 504. Turn left and travel southeast 7 miles to the campground.

GPS COORDINATES

Zone 12S
Easting 519412
Northing 3827841
North 34° 35' 31.92"
West 110° 47' 17.94"

25
KNOLL LAKE CAMPGROUND

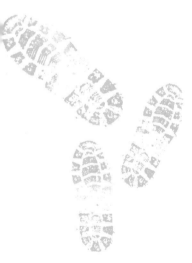

> *Cast a line from the rocky shoreline or bring a small boat.*

THE MOGOLLON RIM IS A SHEER PALISADE of limestone and sandstone cliffs that runs diagonally across much of Arizona, marking the boundary between the Sonoran Desert lowlands and the Colorado Plateau. As you climb northward from the Valley of the Sun, you leave behind the realm of ocotillo and saguaro for a dense forest of ponderosa pine. The dramatic, canyon-carved slopes rise to more than 7,000 feet, and among the trees are scattered springs, streams, and a dozen lakes, making this one of the state's most popular summer destinations. Split between two national forests, the Coconino in the west and the Apache Sitgreaves in the east, the rim country offers a plethora of camping, from primitive, secluded, dispersed sites to RV-friendly recreation areas. Knoll Lake Campground, just up the road from 75-acre Knoll Lake, strikes a good balance, with 33 developed sites nestled among the trees.

As you pull in, look for the bearded mountain man relaxing in site 1. Don't be deterred by the snarling bearskin draped over his chair. Camp host Eddie is very friendly and has a few yarns to spin. He'll set you straight about the hazards of leaving food or personal hygiene products in your tent. As he says, "It's a terrible sight to see a bear stumbling around in lipstick and high heels, although they don't look bad in tights. Of course," he continues with a wink, "I've been up here a long time." In fact, 2007 was Eddie's fourth year at Knoll Lake, working for Recreation Resource Management, a concessionaire that manages many campgrounds in the national forests.

The campground is laid out in an uneven figure eight, with the site numbers increasing as you go counterclockwise. It's nicely organized so that the sites near the entrance (sites 2 through 6 and 33) have pull-throughs or larger parking tabs to accommodate RVs

RATINGS

Beauty: ✿ ✿ ✿
Privacy: ✿ ✿ ✿
Spaciousness: ✿ ✿ ✿ ✿
Quiet: ✿ ✿ ✿
Security: ✿ ✿ ✿
Cleanliness: ✿ ✿ ✿ ✿ ✿

and trailers, and the rest of the well-spaced sites better suit tent campers. Major renovations in 2006 left all campsites with cleared, leveled tent pads, nice concrete picnic tables, standing grills, and fire rings. Several sites offer two tent pads and two picnic tables. The larger loop circles a small hill, so sites inside the loop are up on the hillside and sites outside the loop are set below or away from the road. Sites 20 (a double) and 18 are well below the road, with stone stairs leading down to them. These sites feel much more secluded and private. Sites 23 through 25 are on the edge of their own loop and spacious enough for larger groups.

Knoll Lake Campground fills up during the summer season and occasionally gets folks who've come to party by firelight, but for the most part the campers are families up to enjoy the cool water and great scenery. Knoll Lake is neither as primitive as nearby Bear Canyon nor as bustling as its larger neighbor, the Aspen Campground at Woods Canyon Lake. On weekends the woods are full of dispersed campers as well. The meadowlarks are louder, but you may hear engine noise or the occasional whoop and holler.

The high elevation means cool, comfortable temperatures during summer, but expect heavy rains (even hail!) from July to September during the monsoon season. While driving, keep an eye out for deer and especially elk, which are large enough to completely cover the windshield of your average sedan (don't ask us how we know). The Game and Fish Department, Arizona Department of Transportation, Federal Highway Administration, and the U.S. Forest Service are collaborating on an experimental elk crossing along AZ 260, where the elk are funneled either under or across the road. Where underpasses are impractical, flashing signs notify motorists when nearby animals trigger the electronic sensors.

Just a mile down the road from the campground is Knoll Lake, named for the former hilltop that now forms a small island in its center. Brook, brown, and rainbow trout are stocked here. Cast a line from the rocky shoreline or bring a small boat. The lake is restricted to electric motors only and is favored by people with kayaks, canoes, or kickboats.

KEY INFORMATION

ADDRESS:	Mogollon Rim Ranger District H.C. 31, Box 300 Happy Jack, AZ 86024
OPERATED BY:	Coconino National Forest
INFORMATION:	(928) 477-2255, www.fs.fed.us/r3/coconino
OPEN:	Mid-May–October, depending on weather
SITES:	33
EACH SITE:	Picnic tables, fire ring, upright grills
ASSIGNMENT:	First come, first served; no reservations
REGISTRATION:	With camp host
FACILITIES:	Vault toilets, boat ramp, campground host, water spigots
PARKING:	At sites
FEE:	$12
ELEVATION:	7,400 feet
RESTRICTIONS:	*Pets:* On leash only *Fires:* In fire rings only *Alcohol:* Permitted *Vehicles:* 32-foot length limit; ATVs prohibited *Other:* 14-day stay limit; horses prohibited; off-road vehicles prohibited except to enter and exit campground; 1-horsepower electric boat-motor limit; quiet hours 10 p.m.– 6 a.m.; discharging of firearms prohibited; checkout 1 p.m.

MAP

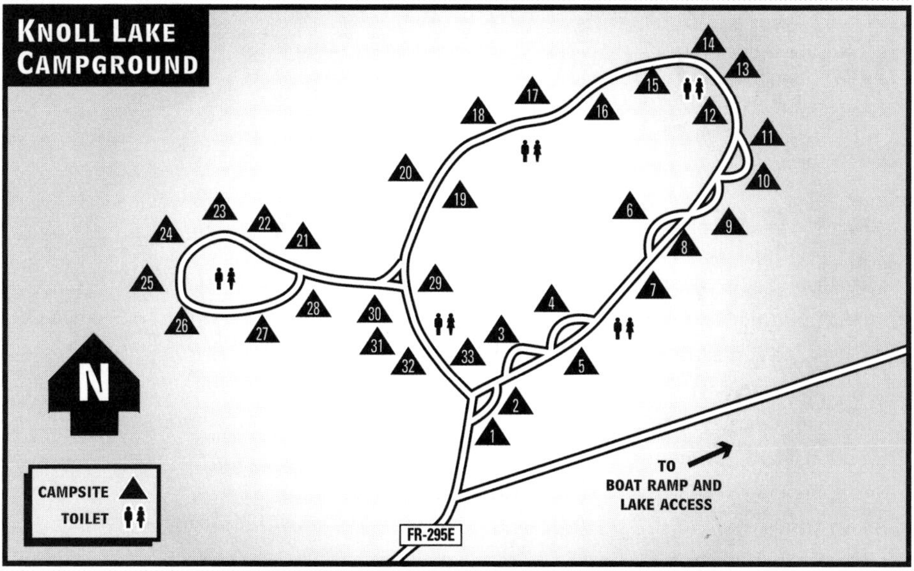

KNOLL LAKE CAMPGROUND
N
CAMPSITE
TOILET
TO BOAT RAMP AND LAKE ACCESS
FR-295E
1
2
3
4
5
6
7
8
9
10
11
12
13
14
15
16
17
18
19
20
21
22
23
24
25
26
27
28
29
30
31
32
33

GETTING THERE

From Payson, take AZ 260 east 29 miles to the Rim Road (FR 300). Turn left and continue northwest 21 miles to FR 295E. Turn right and drive north 3.5 miles to the campground.

GPS COORDINATES

Zone 12S
Easting 491361
Northing 3809370
North 34° 25' 32.76"
West 111° 5'38.46"

Hiking, biking, and riding trails crisscross the area, including a challenging but rewarding stream hike to Fossil Springs near Strawberry. The 100-mile General Crook Trail runs relatively flat along the Mogollon Rim, with spectacular views over Payson and the Hellsgate Wilderness to the Mazatzal and Sierra Ancha mountains. The trail parallels Forest Road 300, a graded gravel route also known as the Rim Road, which can be combined with FR 321, FR 96, FR 95, and AZ 87 to make a 60-mile scenic drive looping through the Rim country. This is an especially good trip to take in the fall when the leaves are changing. Pine and Strawberry, along AZ 87, offer gas, groceries, lodging, and special events throughout the year, and in August Payson boasts the "World's Oldest Continuous Rodeo." For another superlative, see the world's largest travertine natural bridge at Tonto Natural Bridge State Park, just south of Pine.

26
FR 9350
DISPERSED AREA

JUST 90 MILES NORTH OF PHOENIX, after a beautiful drive along the Beeline Highway 87 through the Mazatzal Mountains, you arrive in the old mining and lumber town of Payson. The saguaros have disappeared, replaced by pine trees; the temperature decreases as your elevation increases. This is rim country. The town sits at the base of the Mogollon Rim, pronounced *muggy-own* and named after Spanish governor Juan Ignacio Flores Mogollon. In town, turn right at the stoplight and take AZ 260 east, with the rim looming above you to the north and the Hellsgate Wilderness spreading out below to the south.

The best camping on the rim.

Stop at the visitor center, on the right as you finally top the rim, and talk to the Forest Service rangers and volunteers about the area. On one July afternoon, caught inside during a downpour, we chatted with ranger Paul Schilke, who told us about several designated dispersed camping areas on the Mogollon Rim. They're not currently listed on the Forest Service Web sites, but the rangers will clue you in. Ranger Schilke said the best camping on the rim is on Forest Road 9350, and we agree. Half the dispersed sites along this road actually perch at the edge of the 2,000-foot escarpment, with 180-degree views across miles of mountains and valleys below. In our opinion, the view is second only to the Grand Canyon, and on top of it all, it's free.

To get there, turn off AZ 260 opposite the visitor center, onto the Rim Road (FR 300), passing the turnoff for popular Woods Canyon Lake. On your way, stop at any of the three scenic overlooks to see what's in store for you. Continue 2 miles past where the pavement ends and turn left on FR 9350.

The campsites scatter 1.25 miles along both sides of FR 9350, but you'll find the coveted rim sites to the south. If possible, grab C7, C21, C22, C24, or C26;

RATINGS

Beauty: ✩ ✩ ✩ ✩ ✩
Privacy: ✩ ✩ ✩ ✩
Spaciousness: ✩ ✩ ✩ ✩
Quiet: ✩ ✩ ✩
Security: ✩ ✩ ✩
Cleanliness: ✩ ✩ ✩

KEY INFORMATION

ADDRESS: Black Mesa
Ranger District
P.O. Box 968
Overgaard, AZ
85933

OPERATED BY: Apache Sitgreaves
National Forests

INFORMATION: (928) 535-4481,
www.fs.fed.us/r3/
asnf

OPEN: Year-round if
accessible

SITES: 42

EACH SITE: Fire ring, some
have picnic tables

ASSIGNMENT: First come, first
served; no
reservations

REGISTRATION: None required

FACILITIES: Vault toilet at
trailhead

PARKING: At campsites

FEE: Free

ELEVATION: 7,600 feet

RESTRICTIONS: *Pets:* On leash only
Fires: In fire rings
only
Alcohol: Permitted
Vehicles: No
restrictions; high
clearance recom-
mended for some
sites
Other: 14-day stay
limit; pack in/
pack out;
bear country food-
storage restric-
tions; firearms
prohibited; fire-
wood gathering
prohibited;
10 people per site

from these sites you have your own private scenic overlook and can see the rim drop nearly straight down below you. There, the same tall ponderosa pines that tower over you in camp look like bonsai trees and soon meld into a green, rolling carpet spreading as far as the eye can see.

A few of the rim sites where the road runs closer to the edge are shallow and compact. But if you're willing to sacrifice some view to gain a bit of space, the sites on the north side tend to be large enough for multiple tents and vehicles, and are tucked well back—100 feet or more—from the road. Site C31 sits almost 400 feet back in the trees, but you'll find the best combination of solitude and stunning views at site C36.

After site C38, the road curves away from the rim and the ponderosas make way for oaks and a small clearing. The road is closed at the end of FR 9350, so all traffic must double back, and the last few sites away from the rim will see the fewest passers-by. A numbered fiberglass post at the road marks each site, and another within the site indicates roughly where you should camp. You'll find a stone fire ring and usually a picnic table but no trash service. The only restroom is at the Carr Lake trailhead near the entrance.

Be sure to bring your jacket. Even during tank-top and flip-flop weather in Phoenix, the air is much cooler here at 7,600 feet. The pines, aspens, and oaks shade you during the heat of the day and make hiking pleasurable. Be wary during summer thunderstorms—the rim is said to have one of the country's highest frequencies of lightning strikes.

The Drew Canyon Trail #291 works its way through the campground and drops 800 feet in 1 mile to connect with the Highline National Recreation Trail. The Highline Trail #31, first blazed in the late 1880s, runs 51 miles along the base of the rim. Today it serves as the central hub for an extensive network of trails above and below the escarpment, some of which comprise a portion of the Arizona Trail. Part of the network of trails that traverses the entire state from Mexico to Utah, this section begins near Pine, traveling with the Highline Trail to the East Verde River and up and over the rim to FR 300. Above the rim, the General George

MAP

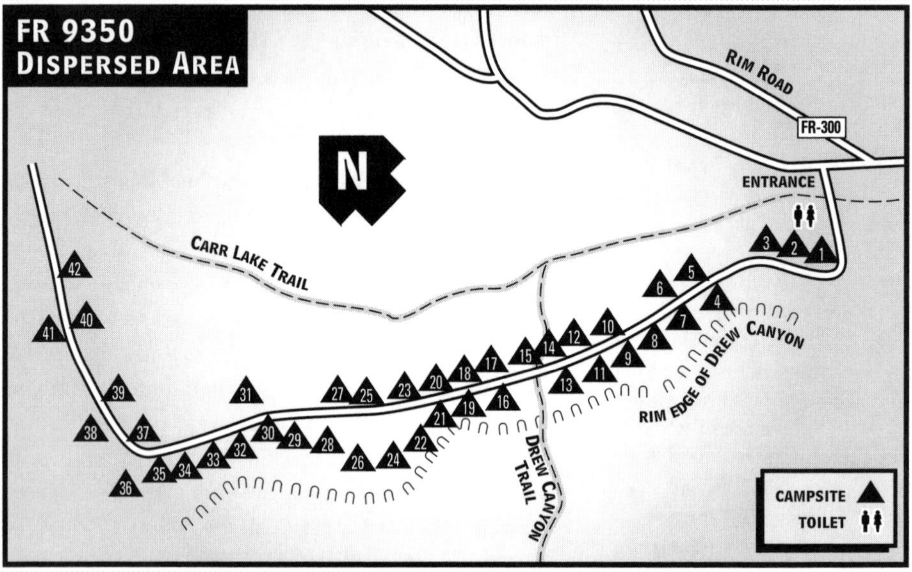
FR 9350
Dispersed Area
Rim Road
FR-300
Entrance
Carr Lake Trail
Drew Canyon Trail
Rim Edge of Drew Canyon
N
Campsite
Toilet

Crook National Recreation Trail travels for more than 100 miles, tracing the route that its famous namesake established as a supply line from Camp Verde to Fort Apache during the Apache Wars. Along the rim it parallels FR 300, but hikers, bikers, and equestrians can follow the chevrons, and even some of the frontier army's remaining blazes, along the original track.

There's a lot more to do and see in the rim country, also well known for its many lakes and streams. For more details, see the Knoll Lake (25) and Chevelon Crossing (24) profiles.

GETTING THERE

From Payson, take AZ 260 east 35 miles to FR 300. Turn left and drive north 5.25 miles to FR 9350. Turn left to enter the campground.

GPS COORDINATES

Zone 12S
Easting 502647
Northing 3799586
North 34° 20' 15.24"
West 110° 58' 16.38"

> *Fool Hollow offers lakeshore views at all campsites.*

REMEMBER WHAT CAMPING WAS LIKE when you were a kid? Remember exploring all of the nature trails and paths that led into the woods, knowing the whole campground was yours to discover? Remember catching that sunfish that was so big that Dad had to help you reel it in? How about the hours spent playing card games in the tent, desperate for the rain to end? Carrying an awkward armful of kindling back to the campsite? Being too impatient to hold your marshmallow over the hot coals and instead burning it in the direct flame? Fool Hollow Lake Recreation Area is the kind of campground where those childhood memories are made.

Lying within the city limits of Show Low, this campground is a perfect getaway for a family vacation. The area shares the tall pines and fine climate of the White Mountain Apache Reservation just to the south, but it hasn't always been a desirable location. When Thomas Westly Adair first settled here to farm in the 1880s, the locals joked that only a fool would try it. Although the town that bore Adair's name was swallowed by the lake in 1956, the area remains Fool Hollow. Opened in 1994, the park is a joint venture between Arizona State Parks, the Apache-Sitgreaves National Forest, Arizona Game and Fish, the City of Show Low, and several corporate sponsors. The result of this collaboration is a well-managed and well-maintained park, nicely designed with smooth, accessible trails and modern facilities, as well as fishing and boating on the 150-acre lake.

A section of the campground at Fool Hollow is designated for tent campers only, on three paved loops named after locally seen raptors: Bald Eagle, Osprey, and Northern Harrier. The loops are arranged so that each of the 31 sites has its back to the east leg of the lake, providing lakeshore views at all campsites. One

RATINGS

Beauty: ✿ ✿ ✿
Privacy: ✿ ✿
Spaciousness: ✿ ✿
Quiet: ✿ ✿ ✿
Security: ✿ ✿ ✿ ✿
Cleanliness: ✿ ✿ ✿ ✿ ✿

official trail and any number of easy scrambles lead down the rocky slopes to the water's edge. The sites lie in a ponderosa, pinyon, and juniper belt, and most have a reasonable amount of shade. While generally compact and quite close together, many of the sites offer enough room to set up a couple of tents. About half of them share a paved parking tab, so you may find yourself in conversation with your neighbors. At 17 and 18 on the Osprey Loop, you'll find true double sites. Site 16 on the Osprey Loop and site 25 on Bald Eagle are designed to be handicap-accessible, as are the shower and toilet facilities. Sites 15, 16, 20, 24, and 31 provide a little more distance from nearby campers.

Each site contains a picnic table, steel fire ring, and standing grill, as well as a cleared tent area. Only sites 29, 30, and 31 are within sight and (possibly) hearing of the campground's RV section. The first-come, first-served sites usually fill up during the summer peak. For a weekend stay, come on a Thursday morning to guarantee a spot. A resident campground host can be found just down the road in the RV section on Mallard Loop, where you can also buy firewood and ice. The park is open year-round, but come prepared for cold nights October through April, and for the usual summer afternoon rains.

The day-use area offers playgrounds, a separate boat ramp, and group ramadas that are available by reservation and can accommodate up to 200 people. They are a popular choice for both local citizens and tourists for family reunions and birthday parties. These facilities sit across the lake from the campground, reducing traffic through the sites. Another playground across from the Osprey Loop provides a safe, enjoyable place for the kids to meet new friends.

Fool Hollow is one of the friendliest campgrounds we've seen for people with limited mobility—even the fishing docks down by the boat ramp are wheelchair accessible. Fishing is the main attraction here, with a large variety of species (including rainbow and brown trout, bass, northern pike, crappies, and catfish) waiting to be lured from the depths of the lake. Regulations allow boats with motors up to ten horsepower. Swimming is not prohibited but not encouraged; no lifeguards

KEY INFORMATION

ADDRESS:	1500 North Fool Hollow Lake Show Low, AZ 85901
OPERATED BY:	Arizona State Parks
INFORMATION:	(928) 537-3680, www.azstateparks.com
OPEN:	Year-round
SITES:	31
EACH SITE:	Picnic table, fire ring, upright grill
ASSIGNMENT:	First come, first served; no reservations
REGISTRATION:	Purchase daily and annual passes at the park office
FACILITIES:	Flush toilets, showers, amphitheater, boat ramp, water spigots, day-use ramadas, campground host, dump station, fish-cleaning stations, fishing docks, playground, firewood, ice, recycling, handicap-accessible sites
PARKING:	At sites
FEE:	$15
ELEVATION:	6,300 feet
RESTRICTIONS:	*Pets:* On leash only *Fires:* In fire rings only *Alcohol:* Permitted *Vehicles:* 45-foot length limit; 14-day stay limit *Other:* Entrance gates closed 10 p.m.–5 a.m.; 10-horsepower boat-motor limit; no glass containers

MAP

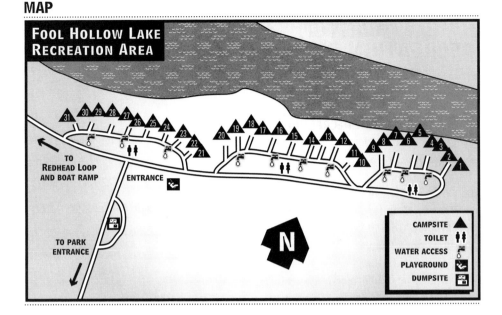

GETTING THERE

From Show Low, take AZ 260 west 2 miles to Old Linden Road. Turn right and drive 0.6 miles to Fool Hollow Lake Road.

or facilities are provided, and watch out for stray fishhooks. The easy trail around the south end of the lake provides terrific bird-watching opportunities, particularly during migrations.

The town of Show Low supposedly got its name from a card game played by two ranchers for possession of the valley rangeland that would become one of Arizona's most pleasant summer havens. Legend says Marion Clark told Corydon Cooley, "Show low and you win," and Cooley cut the cards, coming up with the deuce of clubs (now a civic emblem). Gas, groceries, restaurants, and shops can be found within minutes of the recreation area, and park rangers will give you information on the White Mountains Trail System and other local attractions.

GPS COORDINATES

Zone 12S
Easting 586071
Northing 3792951
North 34° 16' 27.00"
West 110° 3' 53.88"

HAIGLER CANYON RECREATION SITE sits along perennial Haigler Creek, just north of the small ranching town of Young and beneath the Mogollon Rim, the 2,000-foot escarpment that separates the Colorado Plateau from the lower valleys and deserts. The creek is fed by natural springs and stocked with rainbow trout in the springtime. Sycamores, cottonwoods, and Gambel oaks burst into a flurry of color during the fall and early winter.

This campground received a major makeover in 2007. Previously, dispersed camping sites were arranged along the banks of the creek. The renovation resulted in two camping areas outside of the flood channel, significantly reducing human impact on the creek and surrounding vegetation. Near the water crossing, seven sites back the creek bed. The parallel, level parking tabs are evenly spaced 100 feet apart, with oaks, junipers, and a few ponderosa pines growing between. These spots have obviously been created with RVs or trailers in mind, although there's room to set up a tent near the picnic tables. If you want to be as close to the creek as possible, try for sites 2 or 3, which are a little shadier than the others. You should know, though, that better tent sites wait just up the road.

A second area on the opposite side of the road offers seven walk-in sites in the oaks and alligator junipers. Designed specifically for tenters, each has an assigned parking space with its own trail leading to the site. A few extra parking spots are provided, but primarily it's one vehicle per site. Site 8 is the only exception, with pull-in parking similar to the lower sites. All sites consist of level, graveled rectangles with plenty of space for a couple of tents, a fire pit with a grill, and a picnic table with a handicap-accessible overhang on one side. Manzanita and shrub oaks between the sites give them some privacy. Forest Road 200 circles the

> *A major makeover significantly reduces human impact on the creek.*

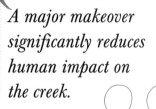

RATINGS

Beauty: ☆ ☆ ☆ ☆
Privacy: ☆ ☆ ☆
Spaciousness: ☆ ☆ ☆
Quiet: ☆ ☆ ☆
Security: ☆ ☆ ☆ ☆
Cleanliness: ☆ ☆ ☆ ☆

ADDRESS:	Pleasant Valley Ranger District P.O. Box 450 Young, AZ 85554
OPERATED BY:	Tonto National Forest
INFORMATION:	(928) 462-4300, www.fs.fed.us/r3/ tonto
OPEN:	Full services April–November
SITES:	14 (7 walk-in tent sites)
EACH SITE:	Picnic table, fire ring
ASSIGNMENT:	First come, first served; no reservations
REGISTRATION:	On-site self-registration
FACILITIES:	Vault toilets, campground host
PARKING:	At campsites
FEE:	$6
ELEVATION:	5,300 feet
RESTRICTIONS:	*Pets:* On leash only *Fires:* In fire rings only *Alcohol:* Permitted *Vehicles:* 16-foot length limit *Other:* 14-day stay limit; bear country food-storage restrictions

campground, coming a little close to sites 8, 9, and 14, but the road rarely receives enough use for traffic noise or dust to be much of an issue. Site 9 sits farther back than 8, and feels nicely secluded despite the road. All of the sites should have some afternoon shade, but 12 and 13 promise cool mornings and evenings; these are our favorite picks. There's a dedicated host site at the tent loop's entrance, across from site 8. Clean, brand-new vault toilets were added to each camping area.

It's a short walk to the creek from the tent sites, but you'll find two nice picnic areas with restrooms much closer to the water. Other perks from the renovation include new trails around the campground, including one along the creek that will allow anglers and hikers to enjoy the beauty of the stream without increasing damage to the fragile riparian ecosystem.

Just a mile up FR 200 is the trailhead for the Bear Flat Trail #178, an old jeep trail that leads into the Hellsgate Wilderness. Hellsgate encompasses 37,440 acres of rugged mountains and steep canyons carved by Haigler and Tonto creeks; at their confluence in a deep gorge is Hell's Gate. The best way to access Hell's Gate is by the Hell's Gate Trail #37. You'll find the trailhead off of FR 405, near Little Green Valley and Ponderosa Campground. Note that the best access is rated at Most Difficult and requires 11 miles of steep climbs and downhill scrambles before reaching the final descent to the water—this wilderness is truly wild and only for the fit and adventurous. As always, motorized and mechanized vehicles are forbidden in the wilderness. You are more than a mile high here and can expect four distinct seasons. The best time to visit is in the spring when the creek will be flowing strongly, or in the fall when you can catch the leaves changing in the Sierra Ancha Mountains. As you drive from the campground to Young, you'll pass by the gravesite of the unnamed Navajo sheepherder who was the first victim of the long-lasting Pleasant Valley War, an infamous feud between the Tewksbury and Graham clans. In Young, long tamed but still a ranching town, you will find two restaurants, a grocery store, a gas station, and lodging. You can reach Haigler Creek easily by coming south from AZ 260, although in places the road becomes

MAP

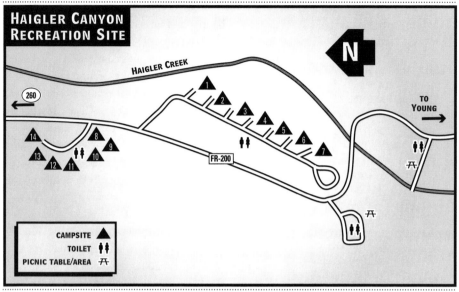

HAIGLER CANYON RECREATION SITE

HAIGLER CREEK

260

TO YOUNG

FR-200

CAMPSITE	▲
TOILET	👫
PICNIC TABLE/AREA	🪑

one lane, hugging tight around blind curves with sheer drops (your passengers will enjoy the view). To enjoy the full beauty of this area, drive the length of AZ 288 from Roosevelt Lake to the rim or vice versa. The Sierra Anchas are some of the most beautiful yet least traveled mountains in central Arizona.

GETTING THERE

From Young, take FR 512 north 3 miles to FR 200. Turn left and drive 9 miles to the campground.

From Payson, take AZ 260 east 24 miles to FR 291. Turn right and drive southeast 3 miles to FR 200. Turn right and continue southeast 5 miles to the campground.

GPS COORDINATES

Zone 12S

Easting 503373

Northing 3786665

North 34° 13' 15.72"

West 110° 57' 48.18"

29
WORKMAN CREEK
FALLS CAMPGROUND

> *Enjoy the Sierra Anchas before the rest of the crowd discovers them.*

THE TRIP FROM GLOBE TO YOUNG along the Desert to Tall Pines Scenic Drive (AZ 288) takes you from the sere valley around Roosevelt Lake to the ponderosa pines, maples, and aspens blanketing the Sierra Anchas. Rounding the southern end of the lake, you cross the Salt River near the Roosevelt Lake Diversion Dam, the end of a day's trip for many rafters on the Salt. As you climb higher you see down the length of 22,000-acre Roosevelt Lake, which looks even larger in its mountainous setting. The road passes many deep side canyons full of sharp pinnacles and hoodoos, then suddenly plunges into sun-dappled forest. From this point, recently laid pavement alternates with smooth gravel.

You soon reach Sawmill Flats, the first of several camping opportunities on the way to Young. The history is reflected in the name, but all that remains now are the "flats" that form this small, dispersed area among tall, second-growth ponderosas. Rose Creek Campground, a few miles on, has six pleasant sites lining an intermittent creek; we especially liked the last, secluded site on the turnaround. With vault toilets, picnic tables, fire pits, and some upright grills, it's a nice place to stay if you'd like a little more "campground" in your camping.

We prefer more-primitive Workman Creek Falls for its perennial stream and deep-canyon feel. Turn down Forest Road 487 and drive 3 miles. You may glimpse an ominous warning sign up a trail near the Elks Youth Camp; there are old uranium mines and dangerous open shafts nearby. In fact, radioactivity levels are too high for overnight camping along a portion of the lower creek, and the Creekside and Cascade areas have been converted to day use only. No need to bring your Geiger counter, though—the Falls Campground is farther up the canyon and away from the mine drainage.

RATINGS

Beauty: ✪ ✪ ✪ ✪
Privacy: ✪ ✪ ✪
Spaciousness: ✪ ✪ ✪ ✪
Quiet: ✪ ✪ ✪ ✪
Security: ✪ ✪ ✪
Cleanliness: ✪ ✪ ✪

The Forest Service claims there are five sites here, but they're not numbered and you'll find only one lonely picnic table. Stone fire rings left behind by previous campers indicate where the likely spots are. The campground is set on a slope alongside the creek, with the first couple of sites just below the road and the rest farther downhill; one set of vault toilets sits roughly in the center. Cliffs rise vertically on the opposite bank, sheltering your camp from chilly wind or oppressive sunshine. The campground is dotted with ponderosa and Douglas fir with a few maples sprinkled in for color. We found a nice, private site downstream where we could hear the gurgle of the creek as we slept.

Once you're settled in, hike or drive the short distance to the spot where Workman Falls drops 200 sheer vertical feet. The falls were barely flowing when we visited in October, but during monsoons or snowmelt they've been described as "thundering." If you drive up FR 487 take advantage of the pullover at the top, where you can walk down and peer (carefully) right over the edge.

Continue on (high-clearance vehicles recommended) and you'll pass trailheads for some of the Sierra Ancha Wilderness's many trails. Wildlife abounds, including elk, mule and whitetail deer, javelina, black bear, and mountain lion. People have also lived here from ages past, and the canyons are scattered with the ruins of generations of cliff dwellings.

A meadow of ferns testifies to ample late-summer rains, and several dispersed camping sites sit in the high, thinning forest. The road eventually leads to the highest point in the Sierra Anchas, 7,694-foot Aztec Peak. The fire watchtower rises high above; from there, you can see all the way to Roosevelt Lake, the Four Peaks, and the Mogollon Rim. Nearby is a mysterious and painstakingly constructed stone living room, where you can sit in two primeval lounge chairs complete with cup holders that face a vast hearth with Arizona as a backdrop.

Heading back to AZ 288 and continuing north, you'll pass over the Honeymoon Divide—another dispersed camping area. Soon you'll see the broad, grassy valley that harbors Young, one of the few true cow towns left in Arizona. Historically, Young is best known

KEY INFORMATION

ADDRESS:	Pleasant Valley Ranger District P.O. Box 450 Young, AZ 85554
OPERATED BY:	Tonto National Forest
INFORMATION:	(928) 462-4300, www.fs.fed.us/r3/ tonto
OPEN:	April–November
SITES:	Approximately 6
EACH SITE:	Fire ring
ASSIGNMENT:	First come, first served; no reservations
REGISTRATION:	None required
FACILITIES:	Vault toilet
PARKING:	At campsites
FEE:	Free
ELEVATION:	6,100 feet
RESTRICTIONS:	*Pets:* On leash only *Fires:* In fire rings only *Alcohol:* Permitted *Vehicles:* 16-foot length limit; no ATVs *Other:* 14-day stay limit; bear country food-storage requirements; pack in/pack out

MAP

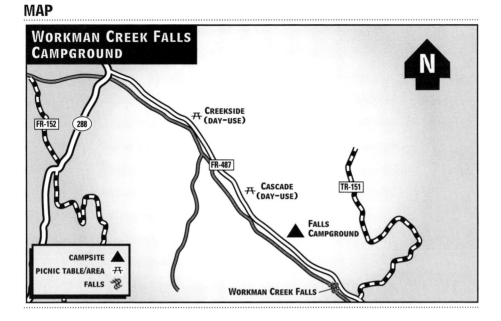

WORKMAN CREEK FALLS CAMPGROUND

N

FR-152 288

CREEKSIDE (DAY-USE)

FR-487

CASCADE (DAY-USE)

TR-151

FALLS CAMPGROUND

CAMPSITE ▲
PICNIC TABLE/AREA ᚛
FALLS ☇

WORKMAN CREEK FALLS

GETTING THERE

From Globe, take AZ 88 north 16 miles to AZ 288. Turn right and travel 27 miles to Workman Creek Road (FR 487). Turn right and continue 2.25 miles to the campground entrance.

GPS COORDINATES

Zone 12S
Easting 505549
Northing 3742673
North 33° 49' 27.36"
West 110° 56' 24.12"

for the Graham-Tewksbury Feud, one of the West's bloodiest and most iconic range wars. Also known as the Pleasant Valley War, it was the raw material for Zane Grey's novel *To the Last Man*. Today Young is still home to working ranches, although you'll see llamas as well as cows. You'll find two restaurants and one gas station in town. If you continue north from Young, AZ 288 becomes FR 512, a graded dirt road with panoramic vistas of the Tonto Basin, which climbs the Mogollon Rim and connects with AZ 260.

Although AZ 288 is now mostly paved, Young residents are divided about finishing the job; some hope for the development and prosperity that's come to towns like Payson, and others would like to preserve the quiet and traditions of this "high lonesome" country. Whichever way it goes, they'll settle it peacefully, but come yourself and enjoy the Sierra Anchas before the rest of the crowd discovers them.

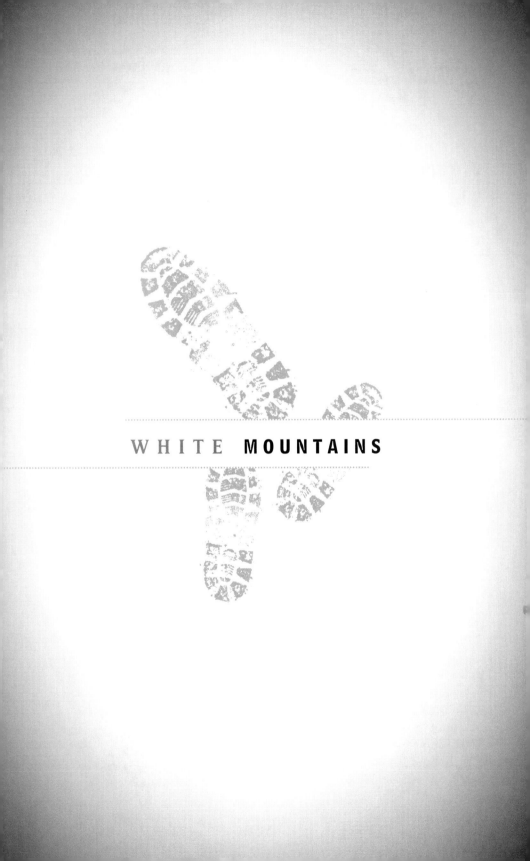

WHITE MOUNTAINS

30
LYMAN LAKE
STATE PARK

NORTH OF THE WHITE MOUNTAINS, the land turns to high desert plains: rolling, grassy hills and nothing for miles but dotted dark shapes resolving into junipers or cows as you approach. A rise or dip in the road may suddenly reveal a rugged wash or outcrop flashing past, then just waving grass, stubby pinyons, and sky again. Hidden back in a rocky bowl in those rolling hills is 1,500-acre Lyman Lake, centerpiece of the oldest recreational state park in Arizona.

As you drive into the park, you pass the dam that creates this reservoir on the Little Colorado River, whose watershed drains the highest northern slopes of the White Mountains, including Escudilla Mountain and Mount Baldy. Look down into the muddy pond to your left and you'll usually see turtles sunning themselves. A former feature of the park was a herd of "wild" buffalo that grazed here, owned by St. Johns Chamber of Commerce and managed by the park. They're sadly gone now, due to lack of funding, but traces of their presence remain on the logo of the general store and on the Buffalo Trail.

Stop at the tiny visitor center on your way in to pick up information on boating and hiking, learn about the park's flora and fauna, browse a collection of books to read and return, or chat about how the fish are biting. Although rangers are often out and about on duty, summer volunteers will assist. Use the self-registration box if the office is closed.

Lyman Lake is the only Arizona state park where you can stay in a yurt–a circular, framed, canvas tent with its origins in Central Asia. The park's four tidy, furnished yurts are a bargain at only $35 a night. You can also rent four cabins that sport porches with lake views and come complete with electricity and climate control.

If you're just fine with your own tent, you'll find plenty of good spots. When you reach the campground,

> *Pitch your tent right on the beach.*

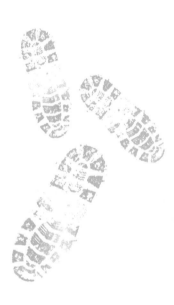

RATINGS

Beauty: ✩ ✩ ✩
Privacy: ✩ ✩ ✩
Spaciousness: ✩ ✩ ✩ ✩
Quiet: ✩ ✩ ✩
Security: ✩ ✩ ✩ ✩
Cleanliness: ✩ ✩ ✩ ✩

turn right to the B and C loops. The B loop has no hookups and consists of five sites among scattered junipers up on the hillside. You can see the lake from here, over the C loop sites. If this suits you, go for B1, a private corner site with a 180-degree lake view. Each B site comes with a small steel ramada shading the picnic table, an upright grill, and fire pit. Tent spots throughout the campground tend to be rocky, but level. The whole area has a wide-open high desert feel, with few trees and a big, big sky.

You can skip sites C18 through C25, where the RVs line up like giant piglets, and head down toward sites C17 through C15. These three sites rank among our favorites, set apart from the rest of the loop with mostly unobstructed views of the lake. You'll discover several more fine sites along the C loop nearest to the lake, as long as you don't mind being part of your neighbors' lake view. For more privacy, head into the D loop. You're farther from the lake here, especially back at sites D34, D36, and D38, but you may find it more peaceful. All of the sites in loop C and many in loop D have solidly built brick ramadas for relief from the glaring summer sun or pounding monsoon rains. They also have hookups, but the park rangers will usually allow tenters to camp at the lower price.

One of the nicest things about this park is that you're allowed to pitch your tent right on the beach below the cabins. Camping used to be available farther along the shoreline, but due to tree damage and waste problems, those areas are now day-use only. The main beach area is convenient to the restrooms, and a ramada and a couple of picnic tables are available for early birds.

KEY INFORMATION

ADDRESS:	P.O. Box 1428, St. Johns, AZ 85936
OPERATED BY:	Arizona State Parks
INFORMATION:	(928) 337-4441, www.pr.state.az.us/Parks/parkhtml/lyman
OPEN:	Year-round
SITES:	56
EACH SITE:	Picnic table, fire ring, some have an upright grill, some have a shelter, some have electrical hookups
ASSIGNMENT:	First come, first served; reservations accepted for group sites, cabins, and yurts
REGISTRATION:	Purchase daily and annual passes at the park office; on-site self-registration when office closed
FACILITIES:	Flush toilets, hot showers, water spigots, boat ramp, beach, day-use area, nature trails, pay phone, yurt, dump station, group sites, resident park manager, firewood, handicap-accessible sites, fish-cleaning stations, fishing docks, ice, general store
PARKING:	At campsites
FEE:	$12; $17 hookup
ELEVATION:	6,000 feet
RESTRICTIONS:	*Pets:* On leash only. *Fires:* In fire rings only. *Alcohol:* Permitted. *Vehicles:* No length limit; ATVs prohibited; 2 vehicles per site. *Other:* Discharging of firearms prohibited; firewood gathering prohibited; checkout time for camping 2 p.m.; quiet hours, 10 p.m.–7 a.m.; removing plants, animals, or archaeological, geological, or historical objects prohibited

MAP

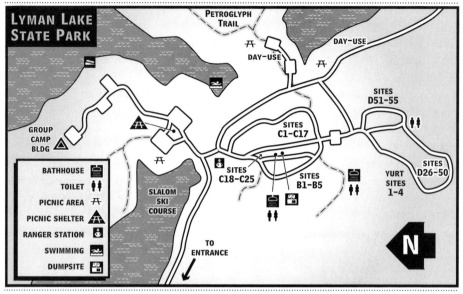

LYMAN LAKE STATE PARK

PETROGLYPH TRAIL

DAY-USE

DAY-USE

SITES D51-55

GROUP CAMP BLDG

SITES C1-C17

SITES D26-50

SITES C18-C25

SITES B1-B5

YURT SITES 1-4

SLALOM SKI COURSE

BATHHOUSE	
TOILET	
PICNIC AREA	
PICNIC SHELTER	
RANGER STATION	
SWIMMING	
DUMPSITE	

TO ENTRANCE

N

Prime time for water sports occurs between Memorial Day and Labor Day, and the park hosts the largest Independence Day fireworks display in these parts. Lyman Lake touts itself as one of the smoothest waterskiing lakes in Arizona and one of the few lakes in the area to have no boat-size restrictions; it even comes complete with its own slalom course. Other parts have been designated as no-wake zones for anglers trying to lure channel catfish and largemouth bass from the depths below.

The park is open every day of the year, and the off-season can be a good time to catch some peace and quiet on the lake. Even if it's too cold to swim, there are plenty of things to do during the cooler months, when the fishing and the hiking may be at their best. Trails include the Peninsula Petroglyph Trail, a 0.25-mile hike up a rocky hill where passing ancients etched numerous signs and symbols into the rock. In season, don't miss the ranger-guided boat tour to an even more spectacular site across the lake at the Ultimate Petroglyph Trail. Guided tours are also available of Rattlesnake Pointe Pueblo, a partially excavated 80- to 90-room village dating from the 1300s.

GETTING THERE

From Springerville, take US 191 north 18 miles to the park entrance. Turn right into park.

GPS COORDINATES

Zone 12S

Easting 648398

Northing 3803593

North 34° 21' 47.04"

West 109° 23' 10.44"

31
LOS BURROS CAMPGROUND

> *If you have the urge to cowboy a bit, you'll find several riding stables in the area.*

IN A LAND OF LAKES AND STREAMS, a campground away from the water can be a quiet oasis. Los Burros is just a few miles north of the bustling lakes of the White Mountain Apache Reservation, but your fishing tackle can stay packed here. Instead, the campground looks out of the tall pines on a lovely grassy meadow. In 1909, the Forest Service set aside 240 acres here for a fire guard, and Los Burros was home to the ranger who rode out every day to man Lake Mountain Lookout, watching for the telltale thread of smoke that would call out brave men to fight forest fires with hand axes and shovels. Later the timber sales agent for the area shared the ranger's quarters, and the meadow and spring served as a camp for lumbermen feeding the mill at McNary, as well as for cowboys and sheepherders moving their stock through the area. Don Hansen, who farmed nearby Reservation Flat in the 1920s and 1930s, remembered one Forest Service employee by the name of Rogers, whose lovely and musical daughters brought an added attraction to the meadow. Les Joslin quotes him in *Uncle Sams's Cabins*: "All the boys in the country knew where Los Burros was."

The historic Ranger Station still stands, awaiting restoration, along with a barn and corral. It has been added to the National Register of Historic Places. The nearby spring is capped now, but the meadow remains, attracting an abundance of wildlife, including black bear, mule deer, pronghorn antelope, and Merriam's turkey. Elk frequently visit here, especially during the fall rut, so listen for the males' bugle call. This is a popular spot for other large mammals as well; horseback riders, mountain bikers, and hikers come to the Los Burros Trail, a 13-mile loop through mixed ponderosa and aspen forest with a moderate elevation change of 500 feet. The trail is part of the White Mountains Trail

RATINGS

Beauty: ✿ ✿ ✿ ✿
Privacy: ✿ ✿ ✿ ✿
Spaciousness: ✿ ✿ ✿ ✿
Quiet: ✿ ✿ ✿
Security: ✿ ✿ ✿
Cleanliness: ✿ ✿ ✿

System, a series of 11 interconnected loop trails in the Lakeside Ranger District built and maintained by volunteers from the community. A short side trip takes you to the top of Lake Mountain and the fire tower, where you can see all the way to the San Francisco Peaks.

Forest Road 224 is graded gravel, but at the turn into Los Burros the gravel gives way to rutted dirt that turns muddy in the late summer rains and spring snowmelt. The managed season is May through October and the road is not maintained for winter travel, although the campground is open year-round for the intrepid and well prepared.

The meadow is on your right as you enter the campground. The three large, open sites closest to the fence best accommodate campers with horses, and two small corrals stand between sites 11 and 12. These sites have great views, if little shade. Spacious site 10 is marked for a host, but Los Burros is not currently hosted. The road forms a rough loop, with sites 8 and 9 and the trailhead at the end. Inside the loop, sites 4 and 7 are a bit overgrown but also have a view, and a nice oak partially shades site 4. The rest of the sites lie inside the tree line and are well shaded. Sites 5 and 6 have sizable tent areas, and site 2 is set back from the rest with some undergrowth for privacy. All have steel fire rings with flip-up grills and metal picnic tables, and there's a vault toilet between site 6 and the trailhead. Parking is at the sites, but trailhead parking on a busy day might encroach on site 8.

The campground is rarely full and mostly used by folks enjoying the cool temperatures or accessing the trail system. When we visited we met a gentleman who spends most of his summer camping throughout the White Mountains with his dogs to get away from the summer heat; a family on horseback with two small children who could have been born in the saddle; and three women who had trailered their mounts all the way from Tucson just to ride the Los Burros Trail.

Los Burros makes a good base camp for exploring the White Mountains and Apache-Sitgreaves National Forest. Unpack your tackle and head south to fish for the native Apache trout, found only in Arizona. Thanks to the conservation policies of the White Mountain

KEY INFORMATION

ADDRESS: Lakeside Ranger District
2202 West White Mountain Blvd.
Pinetop-Lakeside, AZ 85929

OPERATED BY: Apache-Sitgreaves National Forest

INFORMATION: (928) 368-5111, www.fs.fed.us/r3/asnf

OPEN: Full services May–October, depending on weather and road conditions

SITES: 12

EACH SITE: Picnic table, fire ring

ASSIGNMENT: First come, first served; no reservations

REGISTRATION: None required

FACILITIES: Vault toilet, corrals

PARKING: At campsites

FEE: Free

ELEVATION: 7,900 feet

RESTRICTIONS: *Pets:* On leash only
Fires: In fire rings only
Alcohol: Permitted
Vehicles: 22-foot length limit
Other: 14-day stay limit; pack in/pack out; no water

MAP

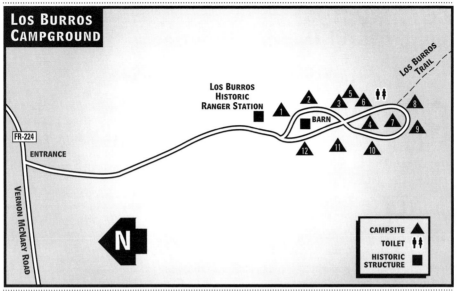

LOS BURROS CAMPGROUND

LOS BURROS HISTORIC RANGER STATION

LOS BURROS TRAIL

BARN

FR-224

ENTRANCE

VERNON MCNARY ROAD

N

CAMPSITE ▲
TOILET 🚻
HISTORIC STRUCTURE ■

GETTING THERE

From McNary, take FR 224 north 7 miles to the campground sign. Turn right and go 0.25 miles to the campground.

tribe, this may soon be the first fish species to be removed from the endangered species list. Stop at the Hon-Dah Resort and Casino for more information about recreational regulations in the Fort Apache Indian Reservation and to purchase permits (for details see profile 34, Pacheta Lake).

Full amenities can be found just to the west in the picturesque towns of Lakeside and Pinetop. The two towns have grown together and have groceries, gas, gifts, restaurants, and rental cabins. If Los Burros has left you with the urge to cowboy a bit, you'll find several riding stables in the area.

GPS COORDINATES

Zone 12S
Easting 612693
Northing 3778980
North 34° 8' 44.34"
West 109° 46' 39.48"

ROLLING, GRASSY HILLS bordered by pines and a wide, blue sky welcome you as you drive windy AZ 261 on the way to Big Lake Recreation Area. The green is a welcome sight for dry eyes used to the desert dust and thirsting for moisture. This is roll-the-car-window-down country, so turn off the air conditioner and let the delightfully brisk summer air whip through your hair. High in the White Mountains in the Apache-Sitgreaves National Forest, 450-acre Big Lake and its smaller sibling, 100-acre Crescent Lake, await with tantalizing cool, blue water.

Big Lake may not be big by other states' standards, but for Arizona it is a respectable size. And besides, it's not the size of the lake that matters, it's the number of campgrounds you can fit around it. By those standards, Big Lake ranks near the top, competing with other biggies such as vast Roosevelt Lake. As we write, Big Lake boasts four campgrounds with another on the way, each named after fish species, mainly trout—the lake's main attraction. The campgrounds vary in amenities and style to appeal to everyone.

When you first arrive, stop at the visitor center if it's open. On our last visit, it had been closed due to federal budget cuts. A phone call to the Ranger Station indicated that it will depend on next year's budget whether public programs will begin again. Whether the visitor center is open or closed, you can pick up the pamphlet for the 0.5-mile, self-guided trail that runs behind the center.

The next left will bring you to Rainbow, the suburban gated community of the campgrounds. You must check in at the entrance station and receive a visitor's pass if you wish to take a tour. Of the four, this is the largest, with 152 sites, paved parking tabs, showers, and flush toilets. As you can imagine, this is where the RVs

> *This is roll-the-car-window-down country.*

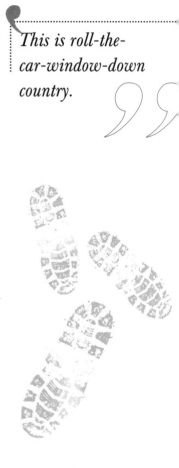

RATINGS

Beauty: ✪ ✪ ✪
Privacy: ✪ ✪ ✪
Spaciousness: ✪ ✪ ✪
Quiet: ✪ ✪ ✪
Security: ✪ ✪ ✪
Cleanliness: ✪ ✪ ✪

hang out. If you prefer a tent spot without an HOA, follow the contour of the lake to Grayling Campground. Designed to appeal to either RVers or tent campers, the campground offers paved roads and sites with pull-throughs or large parking tabs, but they're spread well apart and there are some nice tent spots. At Grayling, like Rainbow, you get a shady site among the trees but no lake view. Your next option is Brook Char. The 12 walk-in, tent-only, reservable sites here are on a hillside, and many have a great view of the lake. The host here takes care of both Brook Char and Cutthroat.

We recommend staying at Cutthroat, the last campground of the four. Once past the Brook Char parking lot, take the next left up the dirt one-way loop. The road is narrow and the parking pullouts small, so you probably won't find even a pop-up trailer here. Most of the sites are on the inside of the loop, on a wooded hillside overlooking Big Lake. Site 3, which is nicely secluded, has its own parking off the road. Outside of the loop, sites 4, 8, and 18 nestle beneath the ponderosas. Site 12 is large and well screened, with no close neighbors. The forest turns to meadow near sites 13 through 17, giving them an open feel and unobscured lake views. Sites 5, 6, 10, and 11 are the closest to the lake, with parking off the main road.

Expect heavy rains and lake-clearing lightning on afternoons in July through September. We've seen rainwater running in rivulets down through the campsites, so keep that in mind while choosing your site and setting up your gear. During the winter, the lake is open to ice fishing, but the roads may be impassable due to snow. Brave souls can reach the lake by snowmobile, and camping is free after mid-October. In season, Big Lake Tackle and Supply offers boat rentals, fishing licenses, souvenirs, groceries, gas, clothing, and tackle and bait.

If you've already caught your allotment of fish, the woods are riddled with trails to

KEY INFORMATION

ADDRESS:	Springerville Ranger District, P.O. Box 760, Springerville, AZ 85938
OPERATED BY:	Apache-Sitgreaves National Forest
INFORMATION:	(928) 333-4372, www.fs.fed.us/r3/asnf
OPEN:	Year-round if accessible; full services mid-May–October
SITES:	18
EACH SITE:	Picnic table, fire ring
ASSIGNMENT:	First come, first served; reservations available online at www.recreation.gov or by calling (877) 444-6777
REGISTRATION:	With camp host at Brook Char
FACILITIES:	Vault toilets, campground host, water spigots, boat launch, boat rentals, general store, hot showers, flush toilets, dump station nearby, interpretive activities and programs
PARKING:	In designated spots
FEE:	$12
ELEVATION:	9,000 feet
RESTRICTIONS:	*Pets:* On leash only. *Fires:* In fire rings only. *Alcohol:* Permitted. *Vehicles:* No RVs or trailers; 1 vehicle per site. *Other:* 14-day stay limit; 10-horsepower boat-motor limit; bear-country food-storage requirements; firearm use prohibited

MAP

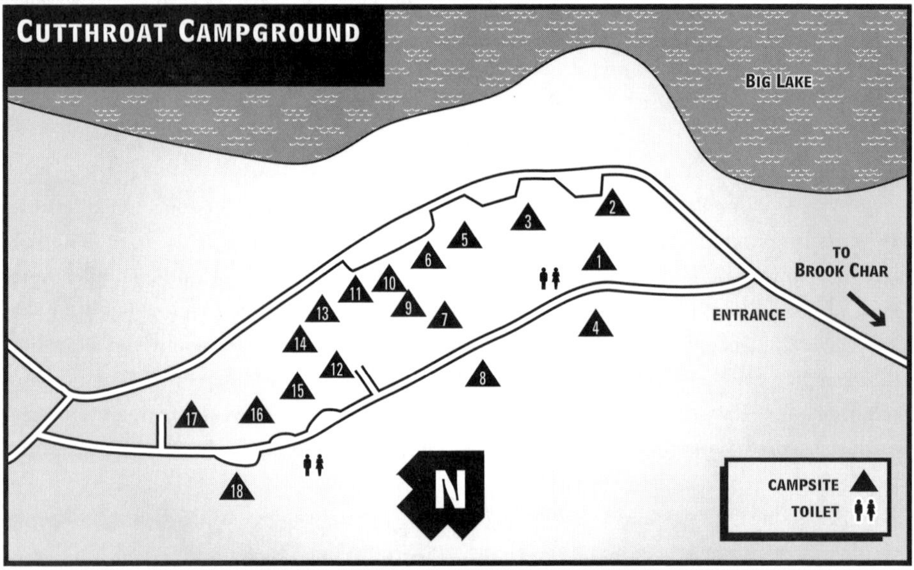

CUTTHROAT CAMPGROUND
BIG LAKE
TO BROOK CHAR
ENTRANCE
N
CAMPSITE
TOILET

explore. Indian Springs Trail #627 starts from loop D of the Rainbow Campground and travels along an old railway line, making a 7.5-mile loop alternating between cool pine forests and wildflower-dappled meadows. A mile-long spur trail leads to the Big Lake fire lookout tower. The tower is usually staffed in the summer, so ask the lookout if you can climb up and enjoy the view. Another spur leads to the West Fork Trail #628, which eventually takes you along the West Fork of the Black River—one of the most beautiful areas in Arizona.

Nearby Mt. Baldy rises to 11,403 feet, and hiking up East Baldy Trail #95 or West Baldy Trail #94 provides unparalleled vistas. The East Baldy Trail starts at Gabaldon Campground and follows the East Fork of the Little Colorado River; the West Baldy Trail starts at Sheep's Crossing and follows the West Fork of the Little Colorado River. The summit itself is on White Mountain Apache land and is closed to nontribal members.

GETTING THERE

From Eagar, take AZ 260 west 3 miles to AZ 261. Turn left and go south 18 miles to FR 115. Turn right and continue 2 miles to the campground.

GPS COORDINATES

Zone 12S
Easting 646454
Northing 3749439
North 33° 52' 30.48"
West 109° 24' 59.40"

33
EAST FORK
RECREATION AREA

> *Spend the day fishing along the banks of the Black River.*

CLOSE YOUR EYES AND THINK OF ARIZONA. What image comes to mind? If you imagined barren wastelands and saguaro cacti, pack your bags and call in sick, because we have something else to show you! In the heart of the White Mountains runs the Black River, a perennial tributary of the Salt River. It waters a forested Eden reached by driving north of Alpine, up the Coronado Highway. You plunge into the midst of Apache-Sitgreaves National Forest, more than 2 million acres of some of the most beautiful land in the state. Once you reach the recreation area, Forest Road 276 runs with the Black River for 6 miles through a deep gorge in the pine-covered cliffs. Rock formations stained with lichen jut out between moss-draped trees, attesting to the rare abundance of moisture here. The river runs fast and clear, racing you down the road.

You can choose among six campgrounds in the East Fork Recreation Area, each within sight or sound of the river. Following a national trend to reduce campers' impact on water sources, some sites have been moved across the road, but no site in all of East Fork is more than a short walk from the stream. Former campground sites have become day-use areas where you may pull off to spend the day fishing along the banks. Trout, smallmouth bass, and catfish all await you in the cold, rushing water. Diamond Rock, named for the distinctive rock formation just down the road, offers 12 sites in three loops. In the first loop, sites 1 through 6 line the river as it meanders away from the road. Dense brush guards the riverbanks here, but that won't slow a true fisherman down. Our favorite site here is number 6, at the end of the loop. Sites 7 and 8 are in the second loop, tucked back into the woods, well separated from each other. You can find a few of the Adirondack shelters originally built by the Civilian Conservation Corps

RATINGS

Beauty: ✩ ✩ ✩ ✩
Privacy: ✩ ✩ ✩
Spaciousness: ✩ ✩ ✩
Quiet: ✩ ✩ ✩
Security: ✩ ✩ ✩
Cleanliness: ✩ ✩ ✩

in Diamond Rock: history you might use to stay dry at site 7 when the heavy monsoon rains fall in July through September. The campground host in the third loop maintains the first three campgrounds along the river. Aspen Campground's six sites overlook a bend in the river. Sites 4 through 6 are the nicest here and perhaps the closest ones to the river in East Fork. At Deer Creek, check out site 5, which is very large and on its own little loop with site 6. Raccoon's ten sites sit very close to each other and right along the road, making it the least attractive place to stay unless you're totally focused on fishing.

The largest campground of the six, Horse Springs takes trailers up to 32 feet long. Its two loops—Polecat and Porcupine—wind through a dense pocket of ponderosa pine along a hillside below the road. The host resides at site 6 in the Porcupine loop, and sites 7 and 8 are handicap-accessible with upright grills. Sites 10 and 12 through 14 sit right next to the water. In the Polecat loop, sites 18 through 21 back up to the river, and here 18 and 19 are the handicap-accessible sites. Horse Springs also offers day-use parking and a picnic area for $3, and a group-use ramada for $75 per day or $100 per night.

You've been slowly descending with the river, and soon the canyon opens into a valley. Here the road forks. If you turn left and cross the river, you arrive at the only campground on the south bank—Buffalo Crossing. The 16 campsites line up under the ponderosas near a green meadow filled with irises and red cinquefoils. You can hear the water cascading over small boulders, though you can't see the river through the brush. A short hike downstream takes you to an old bridge and a great view upstream and down. The campground host, Big Jim (aka Santa—you'll know him when you see him), resides here from May through October—or until they come to take the drinking water tanks away. Even if you don't stay, pay him a visit and be prepared to sit and hear a tale or two. The best site here is 16, spacious and close to the river.

If you take a right at the fork in the road, you'll head up to the West Fork of the Black River. This area is equally lovely, a bit less developed, and the camping

KEY INFORMATION

ADDRESS:	Alpine Ranger District P.O. Box 469 Alpine, AZ 85920
OPERATED BY:	Apache-Sitgreaves National Forest
INFORMATION:	(928) 339-4384, www.fs.fed.us/r3/asnf
OPEN:	May–October
SITES:	77
EACH SITE:	Picnic table, fire ring, some have Adirondack shelters
ASSIGNMENT:	First come, first served; no reservations
REGISTRATION:	With camp host
FACILITIES:	Vault toilets, water spigots, campground host, firewood, group sites and day-use ramadas at Horse Springs
PARKING:	At campsites
FEE:	$10, $5/additional vehicle
ELEVATION:	7,500–7,900 feet
RESTRICTIONS:	*Pets:* On leash only *Fires:* In fire rings *Alcohol:* Permitted *Vehicles:* 32-foot length limit; 1 vehicle per site; ATVs prohibited in campgrounds *Other:* 14-day stay limit; pack in/ pack out; bear country food-storage requirements; quiet hours 10 p.m.–6 a.m.; checkout 1 p.m.; discharging of firearms prohibited

MAP

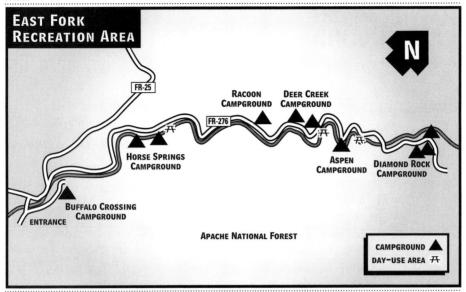

EAST FORK RECREATION AREA

N

FR-25

RACOON CAMPGROUND   DEER CREEK CAMPGROUND

FR-276

HORSE SPRINGS CAMPGROUND

ASPEN CAMPGROUND   DIAMOND ROCK CAMPGROUND

BUFFALO CROSSING CAMPGROUND

ENTRANCE

APACHE NATIONAL FOREST

CAMPGROUND ▲
DAY-USE AREA 🏕

GETTING THERE

From Alpine, drive 2 miles north on US 191 to FR 249. Turn left and drive west 5 miles to FR 276. Turn left and continue south 6 miles to East Fork Recreation Area.

is free. The Forest Service says there are approximately 70 undefined sites here, and undefined is right! A fire ring and sometimes a picnic table are all that mark most of these sites, but you'll find a few Adirondack shelters. To get to some of the sites you need to ford the river—usually possible by passenger car—but be sure to check the water level. To get even farther away from the crowds, follow the remains of the road through the river again to get to the last and least-accessible sites. Campground hosts on each side of the river live here throughout the summer.

GPS COORDINATES

Zone 12S
Easting 657319
Northing 3743239
North 33° 49' 03.60"
West 109° 18' 00.60"

THE APACHE TERM *Hon-Dah* is often translated as "be my guest," and it's an apt name for the small resort town at the crossroads of the Fort Apache reservation. The ancestral land of the White Mountain Apache, the reservation ranges from the stark beauty of the Salt River Canyon to the majestic cloud-swathed peak of Mount Baldy. The tribe welcomes visitors to Arizona's greenest, most hospitable region, a patchwork of forested mountains and blue lakes crisscrossed with perennial streams.

Fishing is one of the region's main attractions, and the campgrounds on the reservation are all associated with one of the many lakes and streams. These areas see considerable use by both visitors and tribal members, but a few more primitive, harder-to-reach areas are seldom busy, one of which is Pacheta Lake.

You'll find Pacheta on the eastern side of the reservation, past popular Reservation Lake and much smaller Drift Fence Lake. You can buy a permit in the summer at the Reservation Lake marina, and you can also rent boats or cabins. The road on to Pacheta begins as a good dirt road that gets considerably worse—four-wheel drive isn't necessary, but a high-clearance vehicle is recommended. Keep your eyes open for loose cattle everywhere on the reservation, even in the campgrounds.

Ponderosa, Douglas fir, blue spruce, and a few aspens surround the small, 68-acre lake. Large boulders covered in lichen scatter on the rocky shoreline, reminding us of northern Minnesota. Camping is restricted to designated areas, but the campsites themselves are not so clearly distinguished. In other, busier reservation campgrounds, tents and small RVs populate any spot that can accommodate them. At Pacheta Lake, the official number of campsites is 15, but we mapped seven clearly defined sites. Each site has a picnic table and a stone fire ring. Signs forbid moving the tables, but you

> *Early in the morning, the trees are reflected i. a perfect mirror of water, with the silence broken only by birdson and perhaps the swish of a fly rod.*

RATINGS

Beauty: ✩ ✩ ✩ ✩
Privacy: ✩ ✩ ✩ ✩ ✩
Spaciousness: ✩ ✩ ✩
Quiet: ✩ ✩ ✩ ✩
Security: ✩ ✩
Cleanliness: ✩ ✩

KEY INFORMATION

ADDRESS:	100 West Fatco Road P.O. Box 220 Whiteriver, AZ 85941
OPERATED BY:	White Mountain Apache Tribe
INFORMATION:	(928) 338-4385, www.wmatoutdoors.org
OPEN:	Year-round; full services mid-May–Labor Day
SITES:	7
EACH SITE:	Picnic table, fire ring
ASSIGNMENT:	First come, first served; no reservations
REGISTRATION:	Purchase Reservation Camping Permit through White Mountain Apache Tribe
FACILITIES:	Vault toilets
PARKING:	At campsites
FEE:	$8 per day per vehicle for camping, $6 per person per day for fishing, $8 per day per vehicle for outdoor recreation permit
ELEVATION:	8,500 feet
RESTRICTIONS:	*Pets:* On leash only *Fires:* In fire rings only *Alcohol:* Permitted *Vehicles:* ATVs prohibited; RVs not recommended *Other:* No firearms; swimming prohibited; no drinking water available; bear country food-storage requirements

will find that some have wandered away to other sites. The latrines are of questionable age and construction, but thoughtfully placed, with entrances facing the woods, providing great views if the door is no longer attached. Gaps between the wooden planks provide good ventilation. Be prepared to BYOTP. There's an informality to the Pacheta Lake arrangements, but you're well compensated for any inconveniences. Some of the sites are along the shoreline, allowing you to park your canoe or kickboat practically in your camp. Early in the morning, the trees are reflected in a perfect mirror of water, with the silence broken only by birdsong and perhaps the swish of a fly rod. Site 1 is generously sized and right on the water. Next around the loop, site 2 sits on the bank above the trickling stream that feeds the lake, and is an excellent site for bird-watching. Up a slope from the lake, site 3 offers a bit more shade and privacy. Site 6 is small, but has a lovely view. Also on the water, site 7 is the most private of all. This area is abundant in wildlife, so practice campsite food safety and be aware that Mexican gray wolves have been introduced in nearby areas of the Apache-Sitgreaves National Forest and are present on the reservation.

Pacheta Lake is stocked with brown and rainbow trout, for catch and release only. You do not need an Arizona fishing license here, but if you don't belong to the White Mountain Apache Tribe, you will need a tribal permit for *any* recreational activity, including picnicking and driving anywhere off the main paved roads. The Apache take the use and preservation of their land seriously—be sure to get the necessary permits and follow the rules. Regulations and permits are available at Hon-Dah Ski and Outdoor Sport, at the tribal office in Whiteriver, at a few stores in neighboring towns, and from Sportsman's Warehouse in Phoenix and Tucson. During the summer, you can buy permits at Reservation Lake Marina, Sunrise Lake Marina, and the Hawley Lake Store. Pacheta Lake is serviced from mid-May through Labor Day. You may camp at Pacheta outside of the season, but you will have to pack out your trash.

For a lovely drive through canyon views and forested mountains, take uncrowded Y55 from Pacheta Lake to Whiteriver, but beware of logging trucks

MAP

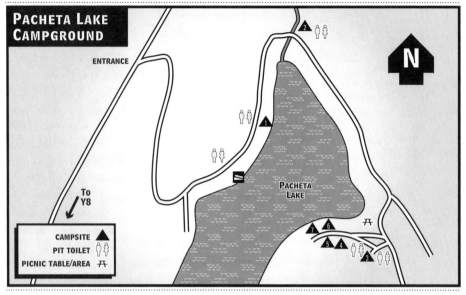

PACHETA LAKE CAMPGROUND

ENTRANCE

N

To Y8

PACHETA LAKE

CAMPSITE ▲
PIT TOILET
PICNIC TABLE/AREA ⊼

during the workweek. Make a stop at the White Mountain Apache Cultural Center and Museum at Fort Apache Historic Park. The White Mountain Apache provided many of the scouts who assisted the U.S. Cavalry during the Apache Wars, and here you can learn more about the tribe's unique culture and history.

If you visit the White Mountains during the summer, you may want to catch a local rodeo. Like many of the Southwest's Native Americans, the Apache are skillful and enthusiastic cowboys. The major event of the year, the Tribal Fair and Rodeo, occurs Labor Day weekend. Summer also offers scenic lift rides at Sunrise Ski Resort, but this playground really comes alive in winter.

GPS COORDINATES

Zone 12S

Easting 634888

Northing 3738608

North 33° 46' 44.46"

West 109° 32' 35.40"

GETTING THERE

From Whiteriver, take Y55 east 40 miles to Y802. Turn left and follow the signs 1.8 miles to the campground.

Alternate route:

From Springerville/Eagar, take US 260 west 3 miles to US 261. Turn left and drive south past Big Lake to FR 249E. Turn right and continue west 5.5 miles to FR 116. Head south 7 miles to the reservation border to Y8. Drive 7 miles southwest past Reservation Lake and Drift Fence Lake to Y802. Turn left and follow the signs 1.8 miles to the campground.

> *Intriguing red sandstone formations appear and disappear as the foliage around you grows more lush.*

THE BLUE RIVER IS COOL AND CLEAR, surrounded by lush greenery, steep canyon walls, tall ponderosa pines, and plenty of history. Driving south on the Blue River Road (Forest Road 281) from Alpine, you descend on dirt switchbacks, following the river over a series of one-lane bridges that gradually lengthen as the canyon grows deeper. Intriguing red sandstone formations appear and disappear as the foliage around you grows more lush. The tall pines linger, but the canyon floor becomes the domain of willows and wild grapes. The road is graded and quite smooth, with a few tight squeezes and curves. During rainy seasons, the road may be muddy, with rocks, branches, or other debris washed down from the upper slopes. Passenger cars should be fine except in very wet or icy conditions.

Some miles of the road make you feel as if you're really traveling into the wilderness, but suddenly a mailbox will appear incongruously by a dirt drive. As the canyon opens into a small, green valley, it's hard not to envy the people who have been lucky enough to live here. The Blue River once flowed through this community with enough force to float logs down to the mining town of Clifton, but the river has dwindled over the last century, and since the Forest Service began a concerted effort to reduce overgrazing, many of the ranches have gone out of business. Signs by the road, however, still invite you to help the Blue River Cowbelles, a local group of ranch women, to keep the valley clean, safe, and beautiful.

Blue, Arizona, now borders Blue Range Primitive Area, 173,762 acres of wilderness accessible by hiking or horseback riding only. Contact the Forest Service for information on the area's many trails. The Blue River is no longer stocked, but you can find wild brown and rainbow trout during spring and fall. The endangered

RATINGS

Beauty: ✪ ✪ ✪ ✪
Privacy: ✪ ✪ ✪ ✪ ✪
Spaciousness: ✪ ✪
Quiet: ✪ ✪ ✪ ✪
Security: ✪ ✪ ✪
Cleanliness: ✪ ✪ ✪

Mexican gray wolf has been reintroduced in the Blue Range area, and many other animals, especially elk, thrive here.

The Upper Blue Campground, 14 miles south of Alpine, consists of just three sites on a small loop among alligator junipers and Gambel oak. At two of the sites, the Forest Service has restored the log Adirondack shelters built by the Civilian Conservation Corps (CCC) during the Great Depression. This is a pleasant area, but you're a little separated from the river here. Past Upper Blue, the vegetation gets thicker and more lush. You pass through more private property, so don't look for dispersed camping along FR 281, and keep your eyes open for loose cattle. On your left shortly before you reach the intersection with FR 567 is the one-room Blue School.

Following the signs, take a right on FR 567 and ford the river. Note the depth marker—and use good judgment trying to cross! The turnoff to Blue Crossing Campground is just past the ford on the right, and a short drive takes you back into a shady four-site loop. As at Upper Blue, you'll find no amenities beyond picnic tables, steel fire rings, vault toilets, and a couple of log lean-tos. The first site, while quite open to the road, has a nice arrangement of CCC shelter, table and fire pit, and a large, flat area under the trees. Site 2 is smaller and closer to the road with barely a pulloff for parking, but also has a shelter with a medium-sized tent area next to it. Check out the original massively built wooden CCC picnic table. Site 3 has good parking, a large, shady tent area, and some screening, and you can clearly hear the stream just a short walk behind you. Site 4, at the end of the tiny parking loop, is shallow and open but has a couple of flat tent spots.

Between sites 3 and 4 you can see the stone steps that were the original entrance, with one of several interpretive signs around the campground. A short trail here leads to a jeep road that takes you along the riverbed. On the other side of site 4 is another short trail that leads through a gate to a rocky outcropping with mysterious symbols pecked into the surface. The Mogollon people left these petroglyphs more than 700 years ago, and although their meaning is now lost, they

ADDRESS:	Alpine Ranger District P.O. Box 469 Alpine, AZ 85920
OPERATED BY:	Apache-Sitgreaves National Forest
INFORMATION:	(928) 339-4384, www.fs.fed.us/r3/asnf
OPEN:	May–October
SITES:	4
EACH SITE:	Picnic table, fire ring, some have Adirondack shelters
ASSIGNMENT:	First come, first served; no reservations
REGISTRATION:	None required
FACILITIES:	Vault toilets
PARKING:	At campsites
FEE:	Free
ELEVATION:	5,800 feet
RESTRICTIONS:	*Pets:* On leash only *Fires:* In fire rings only *Alcohol:* Permitted *Vehicles:* 16-foot length limit *Other:* 14-day stay limit; pack in/pack out; mountain bikes prohibited in the Blue Range Primitive Area; bear country food-storage requirements; no drinking water available

MAP

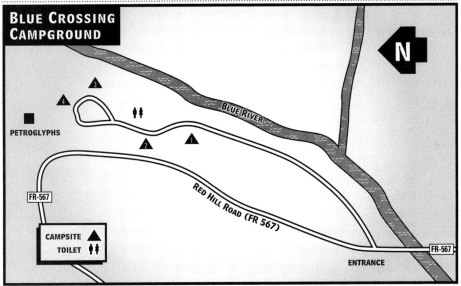

BLUE CROSSING CAMPGROUND

N

BLUE RIVER

3

4

PETROGLYPHS

2

1

FR-567

RED HILL ROAD (FR 567)

CAMPSITE ▲
TOILET ♀♂

FR-567

ENTRANCE

GETTING THERE

From Alpine, take US 180 east 4 miles to FR 281. Turn right and drive south 23 miles to FR 567. Turn right, cross the river, and turn right into the campground.

From Hannagan Meadow, take US 191 north 7 miles to FR 567. Turn right and travel southeast 13 miles to the campground.

GPS COORDINATES

Zone 12S
Easting 676420
Northing 3722522
North 33° 37' 40.44"
West 109° 5' 52.80"

still speak to us about the long history of habitation in this green valley.

An alternate route into Blue Crossing—FR 567, also known as Red Hill Road—climbs steeply out of the valley from the river to intersect US 191, just a few miles north of Hannagan Meadow. A beautiful drive with stunning views of the Blue Range Primitive Area, this route is not for the faint of heart or those with a short attention span. Drive carefully and avoid it in tricky weather. During wet seasons and particularly the spring snow melt, check with the Forest Service for conditions on the road and the river crossing. For more details on the Hannagan Meadow area, see profile 36, KP Cienega Campground.

36
KP CIENEGA CAMPGROUND

TINY KP CIENEGA IS OUR FAVORITE campground in one of our favorite parts of Arizona. Whether you are traveling north from the mining town of Clifton or south from Alpine, you are driving through some of the finest scenery you'll see anywhere. This route, steeped in history and superstition, has been designated the Coronado Trail Scenic Byway, and it roughly follows the northward route of Spanish explorer Francisco Vásquez de Coronado. He and his army passed this way in 1540—the first Europeans to do so—looking for the fabled Seven Cities of Cibola. Coronado never found his cities of gold, but his expedition created a legacy integral to the history of the Southwest.

Possibly the least-traveled and curviest federal highway in the nation, this road rises more than 6,000 feet in elevation over the course of 120 miles through nearly 500 switchbacks—bring your Dramamine. It was once nicknamed the Devil's Highway thanks to its original numbering: US 666. To placate fearful travelers, appease local residents, and prevent the highway signs from being stolen, the highway was officially renumbered 191 in Arizona. Don't let the superstitions scare you. Looking out at the silhouettes of the White Mountains fading into the distance, you feel more like you're headed for heaven.

The word *cienega* means "wetlands" or "marsh," and you pass a small, marshy pond as you make your way to five campsites underneath a small stand of ponderosa, spruce, and Douglas fir. The campground is set a mile back from the highway in a serene meadow. Look for wild turkey, elk, and deer on your way in. On rare occasions, bear and even recently reintroduced Mexican gray wolves have wandered into the campground. Dainty Franciscan bluebells and wild roses line the campground road, and Richardson's geraniums and

> *The campground is set a mile back from the highway in a serene meadow.*

RATINGS

Beauty: ☆ ☆ ☆ ☆ ☆
Privacy: ☆ ☆ ☆ ☆
Spaciousness: ☆ ☆ ☆
Quiet: ☆ ☆ ☆ ☆
Security: ☆ ☆ ☆
Cleanliness: ☆ ☆ ☆

KEY INFORMATION

ADDRESS: Alpine Ranger District P.O. Box 469 Alpine, AZ 85920

OPERATED BY: Apache-Sitgreaves National Forest

INFORMATION: (928) 339-4384, www.fs.fed.us/r3/asnf

OPEN: Full services May–September, depending on weather and road conditions

SITES: 5

EACH SITE: Picnic table, fire ring

ASSIGNMENT: First come, first served; no reservations

REGISTRATION: None required

FACILITIES: Vault toilets, campground host

PARKING: At sites

FEE: Free

ELEVATION: 9,000 feet

RESTRICTIONS: *Pets:* On leash only *Fires:* In fire rings only *Alcohol:* Permitted *Vehicles:* 16-foot length limit *Other:* 14-day stay limit; pack in/pack out; bear country food-storage requirements; mountain bikes prohibited in Blue Range Primitive Area; no drinking water available

towering Jacob's ladder dot the meadow. A picturesque cattle chute stands nearby, left over from the days when the area served as summer pasture for the YY Cattle Company. Look for the small plaque near the entrance to the campground honoring ranchers Toles and Lou Ella Cosper, whose relatives still meet here every June for a family reunion.

Site 1 is the first one inside the small loop, a nicely shaded spot under the pines with a good view of the meadow for watching elk graze at dusk. On the outside, site 2 is compact, grassy, and open, with a pleasant view into the upper meadow. Site 3 is set back toward the trees and a little more secluded. At the back of the loop, site 4 sits up on a slight hill, also in the trees, and has a nicely shaded tent area with no meadow view. As you round the end of the loop, you come to the restrooms and site 5, which is occupied by the camp host during the summer. This is a pull-through inside the loop with room for a trailer and a nice view down the length of the meadow.

All sites have picnic tables, fire rings with flip-up grills, and cut logs for sitting or setting. The campground is open year-round but may be inaccessible due to snow. This area usually gets Arizona's first and last snowfall, and temperatures can get down to the low 30s by October. At nearly 9,000 feet elevation, it is always cool in the summer. You should also be prepared for daily monsoon rains July through September. This lush forest, though blessed with the state's highest rainfall, is plagued by frequent fires and usually has at least one significant forest fire each year, so watch the fire news and obey restrictions!

Spectacular hiking trails crisscross the Blue Range area of the White Mountains. The KP Cienega Trail starts at the campground and quickly descends into a canyon, crossing the KP Creek several times. A nice day hike takes you 3 miles down to the confluence where the north and south forks of KP Creek merge to form two ten-foot waterfalls. If you continue past the falls, you can follow the creek on its journey to the Blue River by combining the hike with the Steeple Trail #73.

KP Cienega is normally full on weekends and often weekdays during the late spring and summer. If

MAP

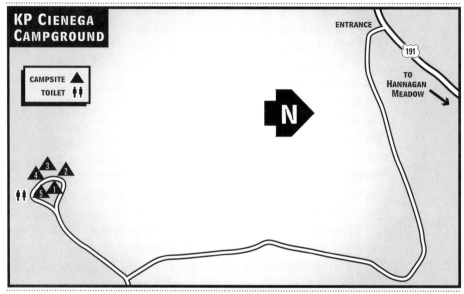

KP CIENEGA CAMPGROUND

ENTRANCE

191

TO HANNAGAN MEADOW

CAMPSITE ▲
TOILET ♀♂

N

you can't find a spot, head just up US 191 to Hannagan Campground. Although larger and more RV-friendly, it's beautifully forested and well maintained. Nearby Hannagan Meadow Lodge offers room and cabin rentals and runs a general store with gas, simple groceries, and souvenirs. The small restaurant primarily serves lodge guests, but if you'd like a pleasant home-cooked meal, call or stop in and make a reservation ahead of time so they'll know how much food to prepare. Innkeepers Diane and Craig Service handle the reception duties as well as serve as waitress and cook. Bill McClain, the lodge wrangler, guides horseback-riding tours and often swings through the dining room in the evening to swap stories with the guests. The lodge porch is a great place to watch the hummingbirds and spy on elk grazing serenely at dawn or dusk in Hannagan Meadow.

GETTING THERE

From Alpine, take US 191 south 27 miles. Turn left at the KP Cienega sign and head east 1.3 miles to the campground.

GPS COORDINATES

Zone 12S

Easting 652191

Northing 3717280

North 33° 35' 03.78"

West 109° 21' 36.06"

37

Clifton

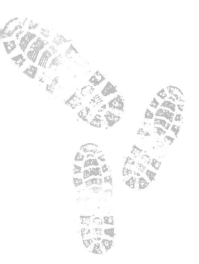

You'll hardly see another soul while in camp.

PICTURE THE PROUD GROOM and blushing bride (hopefully no longer in trousseau), rattling up and down precipitous mountain curves and fording cold running streams, headed for the middle of nowhere to celebrate their wedding night to the music of wind-rushed leaves and murmuring water.

Apparently, that was one forest ranger's idea of the perfect honeymoon. If you agree, follow the ribbon of Upper Eagle Creek as it winds its way through the White Mountains to find this tiny gem of a campground.

From Clifton, take the Devil's Highway (the Coronado Trail) north to Forest Road 217. The beauty of the Coronado Trail always makes me forget how curvy the road is until I glance down and my stomach lurches into my throat. Don't let the thick black line on the map fool you, either: 25 mph is as fast as you'll want to take this highway, so plan accordingly. Once you turn on to Upper Eagle Creek Road, the surface turns to dirt, easily passable in a sedan as long as the roads are dry and the creek isn't running high. The 22-mile road climbs up and down through pinyon-juniper forest and into grassy plains, following sycamore-lined Eagle Creek. At least a dozen "Do not cross when flooded" signs decorate the roadside, half of which are followed by the 15-foot-wide rocky stream. You pass several working ranches (and yes, that cow in front of you *does* own the road), and the Eagle School, which no longer holds classes but still serves as a community hall and polling place. As the road climbs and the valley narrows, the foliage grows more lush.

Just before the road ends at the Four Drag Ranch, the Honeymoon Campground appears on your left. The three sites you see are right along the road, but you won't find that the traffic keeps you up at night. More likely, you'll hardly see another soul while in camp, which is part of the allure.

RATINGS

Beauty: ✪ ✪ ✪ ✪
Privacy: ✪ ✪ ✪ ✪ ✪
Spaciousness: ✪ ✪ ✪ ✪
Quiet: ✪ ✪ ✪ ✪
Security: ✪ ✪ ✪
Cleanliness: ✪ ✪ ✪

The sites are not signed, but there are four picnic tables with associated fire pits that we've numbered from south to north. The first two are within sight of each other under a canopy of sycamore, cottonwood, maple, pinyon, and juniper trees. You won't find designated pads, but plenty of flat earth will easily accommodate large tents. A set of pit toilets with a handicap-accessible concrete ramp separates the first two sites from the third. Site 3, a cul-de-sac with its back to a dry wash, is every bit as large and shady as the first two and affords even more privacy. All three sites are just across the road from the creek, but the bank in this area is reinforced with rough rock riprap that makes for uncertain footing. Stroll 100 yards in either direction and you can more easily reach the river's edge for some fine fishing.

At first glance, this appears to be the extent of the campground, but if you continue down FR 217 nearly to the ranch gate, you'll find one more campsite—this time on the creek side of the road. An immense Arizona sycamore shades the spacious site, whose only neighbors are the infrequent visitors to the nearby trailhead. As at the other sites, you have a picnic table and a metal fire ring with a flip-up grill, and it's a moderate 200-yard walk back to the toilets. This is our pick of the sites.

The campground is open year-round, but the Forest Service indicates its season is May through September. Be prepared for afternoon rainstorms July through September and high water during the spring snowmelt. Fall is a particularly nice time to visit, when the maples and sycamores turn crimson and gold. The only time you might find a crowd here would be during hunting seasons. The forest abounds with mule deer, elk, black bears, and wild turkeys. Eagles do soar here, and herons will fish the creek with you.

Along the same fence line as the ranch gate you'll find the trailhead. Beyond the vehicle gate is FR 8369, an extremely primitive road that is closed from February 1 through June 30 each year. One glance at the yard-deep ruts leading into the creek convinced us we wouldn't attempt this path in anything other than a Jeep or ATV. From here you can access a network of hiking trails, including Squirrel Canyon #34, East Eagle

KEY INFORMATION

ADDRESS:	Clifton Ranger District 397240 AZ 75 Duncan, AZ 85534
OPERATED BY:	Apache-Sitgreaves National Forest
INFORMATION:	(928) 687-1301, www.fs.fed.us/r3/asnf
OPEN:	Year-round if accessible; season: May through September
SITES:	4
EACH SITE:	Picnic table, fire ring
ASSIGNMENT:	First come, first served; no reservations
REGISTRATION:	None required
FACILITIES:	Vault toilets
PARKING:	At campsites
FEE:	Free
ELEVATION:	5,400 feet
RESTRICTIONS:	*Pets:* On leash only *Fires:* In fire rings only *Alcohol:* Permitted *Vehicles:* 16-foot length limit *Other:* 14-day stay limit; pack in/pack out; bear country food-storage restrictions; discharging of firearms prohibited; no drinking water available

MAP

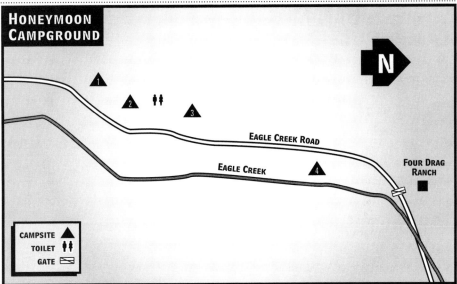

HONEYMOON CAMPGROUND

N

EAGLE CREEK ROAD

EAGLE CREEK

FOUR DRAG RANCH

CAMPSITE ▲
TOILET
GATE

GETTING THERE

From Clifton, take US 191 north 30 miles to FR 217. Turn left and go west 22 miles to the campground.

#33, and Robinson Mesa Trail #27. Trail #33 travels a relatively flat 12.6 miles along East Eagle Creek and eventually lands you at US 191; you can use it as a connector to the Eagle National Recreation Trail, which works its way north from a point on FR 217, touches the highway near Rose Peak, and climbs north to the eastern point of the Bear Wallow Wilderness. Be sure to get information and maps from the Clifton Ranger District before heading out on any of the trails. The Eagle Creek Road runs very close to the San Carlos Apache Reservation boundary, so if you decide to strike out to the west make sure you have any permits you might need.

GPS COORDINATES

Zone 12S
Easting 641051
Northing 3704792
North 33° 28' 23.94"
West 109° 28' 55.14"

38
LOWER JUAN MILLER CAMPGROUND

DRIVE US 191 NORTH through the eastern part of the state and you're exposed to a slice of the vast diversity that makes up the state of Arizona. The road rises from the scrubby floor of the San Simon Valley into the heart of Arizona's copper country. As you climb, you pass through the vast, open-pit copper mines of Morenci and Clifton. The mountains have been transformed into inverted pyramids of marbled horizontal shelves. It's hard not to stare in both horror and awe at the raw kaleidoscope of peach, rust, sage, and slate gray. Beyond the mines, you see the mountains as they looked before their minerals were dug out—rugged, rocky hills dotted green with juniper and pinyon pine. The higher the elevation, the lower the air temperature becomes. Soon you can turn off the a/c and roll down the windows; perhaps the fresh air will help the impending motion sickness as you take another sharp turn around the next switchback.

After 27 miles of breathtaking views and heart-stopping drops, which have probably taken more than an hour to navigate, you reach the turn for Juan Miller Road. Two tiny campgrounds patiently wait for anyone willing to come this far to visit. Upper Juan Miller comes first, and the tight stream crossing easily weeds out the unadventurous and the ponderous. Here you find four sites in a tight loop on hilly, uneven ground. The dense undergrowth and lack of good tent spots make this green Civilian Conservation Corps gem far more suitable for picnics than camping.

Continue the short distance to Lower Juan Miller, which has more room to spread out. The campground consists of only four designated sites, but there are also some suitable dispersed areas; it's unlikely you will ever find this rarely used campground full. Mature Gambel oak, ponderosa pine, and alligator juniper provide an emerald canopy over the entire scene, and the bed of

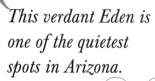

This verdant Eden is one of the quietest spots in Arizona.

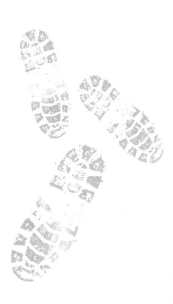

RATINGS

Beauty: ✰ ✰ ✰ ✰
Privacy: ✰ ✰ ✰ ✰
Spaciousness: ✰ ✰ ✰
Quiet: ✰ ✰ ✰ ✰
Security: ✰ ✰
Cleanliness: ✰ ✰ ✰

KEY INFORMATION

ADDRESS:	Clifton Ranger District 397240 AZ 75 Duncan, AZ 85534
OPERATED BY:	Apache-Sitgreaves National Forest
INFORMATION:	(928) 687-1301, www.fs.fed.us/r3/asnf
OPEN:	All year, weather permitting
SITES:	4
EACH SITE:	Picnic table, fire ring
ASSIGNMENT:	First come, first served; no reservations available
REGISTRATION:	None required
FACILITIES:	Vault toilets
PARKING:	At sites
FEE:	None
ELEVATION:	5,700 feet
RESTRICTIONS:	*Pets:* Permitted *Fires:* In fire ring only *Alcohol:* Permitted *Vehicles:* 16-foot length limit; RVs not recommended *Other:* 14-day stay limit; no drinking water available

Juan Miller Creek boasts giant-leaved sycamores. The creek was dry when we visited, but the greenery attests to the abundant moisture available here. In the fall, the leaves create a panorama of gold and russet. Traffic patterns within the tiny campground are hard to discern, but you'll find plenty of places to park. Site 1 has small tent areas close to the picnic table and larger options a few steps away. Site 2 is roomy, but sits right in the middle of the camp area. We prefer site 3, set apart from the others at the end of the line with shrub live oak and velvet ash providing some screening. Shady site 4 backs up to the creek bed and would be very pleasant when the creek is flowing. Be prepared for afternoon thunderstorms during the monsoon months of July through September and for chilly evenings even during the middle of summer.

Arizona has so many lovely campgrounds dating from the Civilian Conservation Corps era that it comes as no surprise to find their handiwork in this verdant Eden, as well. Stonework picnic tables grace each site, along with metal or stone fire rings. There's no host and no water, but bear-proof trash cans and vault toilets are provided. The 16-foot length limit and twisty mountain roads discourage RV traffic. You may find more neighbors here in hunting season than at any other time, since the White Mountains abound with game, including deer, elk, and the occasional black bear or mountain lion. Juan Miller is a quiet place. Catch it without other occupants and you may find it one of the quietest spots in Arizona.

The Juan Miller Road, campgrounds, and creek are named for an early settler who emigrated from Germany and homesteaded in the Blue River area. According to records his name was von Müellar, but locals accustomed to Spanish and English names presumably rechristened him. The road continues 12 miles past the campground, descending to meet the Blue River near the historic XXX Ranch (not what it sounds like to modern ears—that was rancher Fred Fritz's cattle brand). A cold, tumbling trout stream, the perennial Blue is one of Arizona's most beautiful rivers. The isolation of this rare river access makes it a wonderful fishing spot. The Blue is not a runnable river most of the year, but lucky

MAP

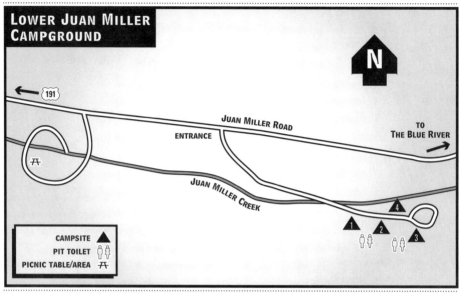

LOWER JUAN MILLER CAMPGROUND

N

← 191

JUAN MILLER ROAD

ENTRANCE

TO
THE BLUE RIVER

JUAN MILLER CREEK

1 2 3 4

CAMPSITE	▲
PIT TOILET	👤👤
PICNIC TABLE/AREA	ᴨ

kayakers with good timing might catch the spring snow-melt. In warmer weather when the water is lower, you can hike upstream toward the Blue Range Primitive Area, 173,762 acres of unmarred wilderness with miles of hiking and horseback-riding trails. Hiking this mountainous terrain is strenuous, since you're either going up or down with every step, but it's incredibly rewarding. This valley has a long history, and with a little exploration you may find evidence of occupation from the heyday of cattle ranching all the way back to Puebloan times.

The Juan Millers also make a good stop before exploring farther up the Coronado Highway. For more information about the area, see profile 36, KP Cienaga Campground, and contact Apache-Sitgreaves National Forest.

GETTING THERE

From Clifton, take US 191 north 27 miles to FR 475. Turn right and go east 2 miles to the campground.

GPS COORDINATES

Zone 12S

Easting 654200

Northing 3682363

North 33° 16' 09.42"

West 109° 20' 39.69"

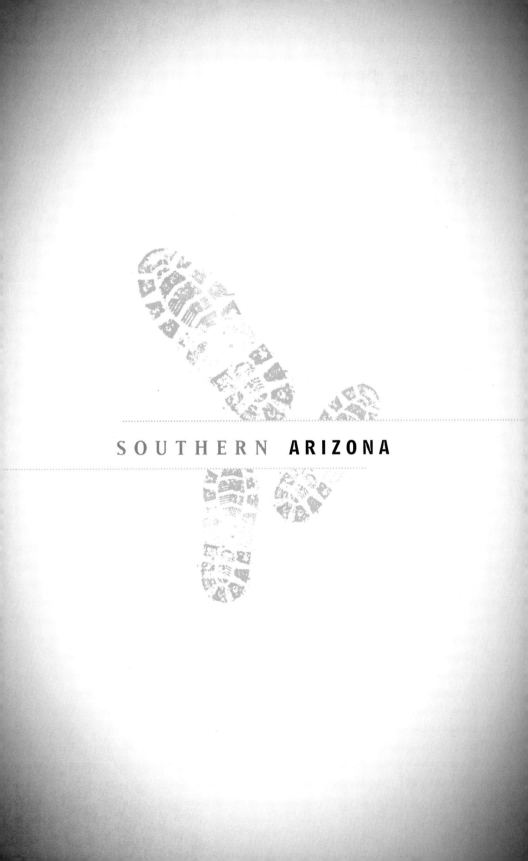

SOUTHERN ARIZONA

39
PICACHO PEAK
STATE PARK

WHENEVER WE DRIVE BETWEEN PHOENIX and Tucson, we always watch for the distinctive shape of Picacho Peak dancing in the distance, marking a rough halfway point. Standing 1,500 feet above the rest of the landscape, this 22-million-year-old lava spike has been a landmark for hundreds of years. Intrepid Jesuit missionary Father Eusebio Kino noted it in the late 1600s, and in 1775 Captain Juan Bautista de Anza passed by en route to San Francisco. The Mormon Battalion, 543 men specially enlisted to fight in the Mexican War, came through Picacho Pass in 1846 on a grueling 2,000-mile trek from Iowa to California, said to be the longest military march in American history. The pass was also the location of the only Civil War battle in Arizona, on April 15, 1862. During the second weekend of March, reenactors in blue and gray take over the park, and you're welcome to come and participate in some living history.

Picacho means "peak" in Spanish, continuing a long tradition of redundant Anglo-Spanish naming that has left Bahia Bays and Camino Roads across the West. Perched on the peak's eastern slope, the park overlooks the vast Santa Cruz flats and the rest of the small Picacho mountain range. After a closure for major refurbishing in summer 2008, the park has a brand-new visitor center where rangers and volunteers will be happy to detail local hikes and history, and provide books, field guides, and souvenirs. Be sure to ask about the interpretive talks held each Saturday afternoon from January to March.

As with all Arizona state parks, the campground is very RV-friendly, with long, level double parking tabs. Never fear, though: several sites allow a tenter to be comfortable away from everyone else, and the presence of electric hookups means fewer generators running (although you may envy the tin-can campers their air

> *For about three weeks the hillsides turn gold and purple.*

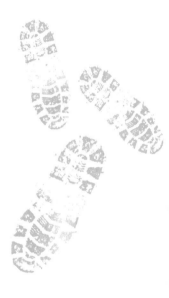

RATINGS

Beauty: ✪ ✪ ✪
Privacy: ✪ ✪ ✪
Spaciousness: ✪ ✪ ✪
Quiet: ✪ ✪ ✪
Security: ✪ ✪ ✪ ✪
Cleanliness: ✪ ✪ ✪ ✪

conditioning). One thing you'll need to resign yourself to is the faint drone and occasional distant whistle of Interstate 10 and its companion railway, which follow the historic route through Picacho Pass.

The campground at Picacho is arranged in three very similar loops, but the park has refurbished loop A for tenters by providing more shade ramadas and turning off the electric hookups; the reduced no-hookup fee applies to only these sites. You'll find our favorite sites outside the loops at the southern end, where a small, craggy ridge rises between the campground and the closest portion of the highway. Paloverde trees and creosote bushes typical of the low Sonoran desert provide some light shade and patchy screening between the sites. Choose one that has a shade ramada if you're visiting during warmer months—June through September daytime temperatures average 100°F. Sites A7 and A11 provide great views of Picacho Peak, but A13 is our favorite, with a ramada, a large, level tent spot, and no close neighbors. If you make it all the way around loop A and find it full, you can also tent in loop B or C at the full hookup price; check out sites B12 and B14, or C11, C17, and C20.

The best time to visit Picacho Peak is in late February and early March. For about three weeks, the hillsides turn gold and purple in an amazing display as the Mexican gold poppies, brittlebush, lupine, and scorpionweed bloom among the cholla, saguaros, and prickly pear. Spring and fall are the park's peak seasons, when the weather strikes a pleasant balance between warm days and cool nights. The pass is often windy, especially in spring, so anchor your tent well.

Among the best features of the park are the hiking trails, two of which lead to the top of the peak (3,374 feet). Leave from the trailhead in the Barrett Loop for a 2-mile hike via the Hunter Trail, or start from the far end of the park at the Sunset Vista trailhead for a

KEY INFORMATION

ADDRESS:	P.O. Box 275, Picacho, AZ 85241
OPERATED BY:	Arizona State Parks
INFORMATION:	(520) 466-3183, www.pr.state.az.us/Parks/parkhtml/picacho
OPEN:	Year-round
SITES:	85
EACH SITE:	Picnic table, fire ring, some have an upright grill, some have a ramada, some have electrical hookups
ASSIGNMENT:	First come, first served; reservations accepted for group sites
REGISTRATION:	Purchase daily and annual passes at the park office; on-site self-registration when office closed
FACILITIES:	Flush toilets, hot showers, water spigots, day-use ramadas, nature trails, pay phone, dump station, amphitheater, drinking fountains, group sites, campground host, resident park manager, firewood, handicap-accessible sites, playground
PARKING:	At campsites
FEE:	$12 non-electric; $20 electric
ELEVATION:	2,000 feet
RESTRICTIONS:	*Pets:* On leash only. *Fires:* In fire rings only. *Alcohol:* Permitted. *Vehicles:* No length limit. *Other:* 14-day stay limit; discharging of firearms prohibited; firewood gathering prohibited; quiet hours 10 p.m.–6 a.m.; checkout 2 p.m.

MAP

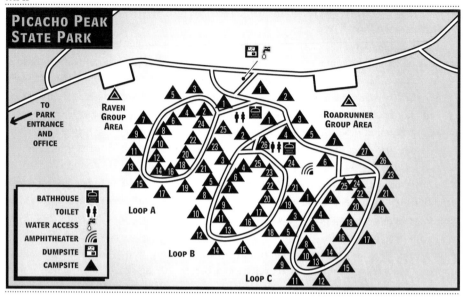

PICACHO PEAK STATE PARK

TO PARK ENTRANCE AND OFFICE

RAVEN GROUP AREA

ROADRUNNER GROUP AREA

BATHHOUSE
TOILET
WATER ACCESS
AMPHITHEATER
DUMPSITE
CAMPSITE

LOOP A

LOOP B

LOOP C

less-steep 3-mile trek. Parts of the trails are difficult; cables have been installed in the rock to aid your ascent. Put your water in a backpack to keep your hands free and consider a pair of gloves. From the peak, the view is panoramic, and soaring turkey vultures exhibit a rare playfulness in the updrafts from the mountain face.

If you aren't up for the scramble to the top, you can hike 0.7 miles on the Calloway Trail to the overlook at 2,274 feet. Branch onto the Calloway Trail from the Nature Trail, a short loop hike that leads you down through arroyos with interpretive signs describing the flora, fauna, and geology of the mountain. Kids are sure to enjoy the playground and the Children's Cave Trail, a short 0.3-mile hike to a small cave with kid-oriented interpretive signs.

Nearby attractions include the Rooster Cogburn Ostrich Ranch, where you can hand-feed ostriches and fallow deer, or be swarmed by rainbow lorikeets. Ostrich keepsakes include feather dusters and eggs (for display or really big omelets). Snack on local pecans and other types of nuts available at the Arizona Nut House, just by the park entrance.

GETTING THERE

From Tucson, take I-10 north 40 miles to exit 219. Follow the signs to the campground.

GPS COORDINATES

Zone 12S

Easting 460796

Northing 3612723

North 32° 39' 05.16"

West 111° 25' 04.92"

THE BEST
IN TENT
CAMPING
ARIZONA

> *The best water hike in Arizona.*

BOXED BY MOUNTAINS and surrounded by wilderness, Fourmile Canyon Campground serves as a terrific base to explore some of Arizona's lesser-known natural treasures. Turn off Pinal Highway (US 70) and onto Klondyke Road. Gravel crunches under your tires as you cross ridged and crumpled badlands between the Pinaleños and Santa Theresa mountains, then descend to the grassy floor of lower Aravaipa Canyon to meet Bonita-Klondyke Road.

Two hopeful prospectors just back from the Yukon gold rush named the town of Klondyke. Although it never yielded the riches of its Canadian namesake, nearby mines dug enough copper, silver, and lead to support more than 500 people. As the mines closed in the 1950s and the profits left ranching, Klondyke's population declined. The sign at the outskirts of town now reads "Pop. 5." The town consists largely of the Klondyke Country Store—a general store, RV park, lodge, and gas station that, sadly, is currently shuttered and up for sale.

At the Klondyke Bureau of Land Management (BLM) Ranger Station, turn left and drive 0.5 miles to the campground. Ten sites are arranged in a valley in the foothills of the Galiuro Mountains. Mesquites 15 to 20 feet tall surround you, providing some shade during hot summer mornings and afternoons. Lighted flush toilets and running water conveniently situated in the middle of the ring of sites add an extra touch of comfort. Undergrowth is sparse, but a bit thicker on the east side in sites 6 through 10. The ground at most sites is sandy and soft, but watch for rocky patches. Each site has a sturdy concrete picnic table, a hearth with a grill, and at least a couple of tent spots. The only exception is site 10, which is better suited for campers who sleep in their vehicle.

For shade and good screening, check out sites 5, 8, and 9, but be aware that if the campground is full you

RATINGS

Beauty: ☆ ☆ ☆
Privacy: ☆ ☆ ☆ ☆
Spaciousness: ☆ ☆ ☆ ☆
Quiet: ☆ ☆ ☆ ☆
Security: ☆ ☆ ☆
Cleanliness: ☆ ☆ ☆ ☆

may get some restroom traffic nearby. If you're with a larger party, sites 1 and 3 combine nicely, and site 7 provides several tent possibilities. Site 6 is nice for dry weather, but watch where you put your tent if the forecast calls for rain. Arizona soil does not absorb water easily. Even a little bit of rain can lead to a lot of runoff. When we visited site 6, you could see where previous rains had left drainage trails through the tent spot.

Outside the loop road near site 6, an overflow area offers extra space, in case you make it all the way to Klondyke and find the campground full. The only time this is likely to happen is during hunting season, when sportsmen flock here to try for mule deer and javelina.

Klondyke is the eastern gateway to Aravaipa Canyon, 42,000 acres of Nature Conservancy Preserve and Bureau of Land Management–designated wilderness, widely regarded among canyoneers as the best water hike in Arizona. Wet-footed hikers enjoy the rare treat of trekking up a spring-fed perennial creek and through an unspoiled natural riparian habitat at the bottom of a deep, scenic canyon. You can hike the 11-mile canyon from one end to the other, or spend a day exploring the side canyons. The BLM issues 50 permits every day—only 20 from the east entrance. Trips are limited to three days (two nights) in the canyon, and reservations can be made three months in advance. Spring and fall are the best times to hike for flora, fauna, and temperature. Fall is particularly beautiful, with the red and yellow leaves of sycamore and cottonwoods reflecting in the clear, blue water. Aravaipa Canyon also forms the seventh segment of the Grand Enchantment Trail, a 700-mile hiking-trail network stretching from Phoenix to Albuquerque.

The ranger at the Klondyke station can fill you in on current road and canyon conditions. An access dispute with a landowner caused the BLM to suspend issuing canyon permits from the east entrance for more than two years (and brought on the demise of the Klondyke Store). While permits are now available again, the dispute continues. Coming in on the main route, be prepared to cross the creek several times before reaching the trailhead. Recent floods have caused a lot of damage along the canyon, making the alternate access route (around the disputed gate) almost impassable and

KEY INFORMATION

ADDRESS:	Safford Field Office 711 14th Avenue Safford, AZ 85546
OPERATED BY:	Bureau of Land Management
INFORMATION:	(928) 348-4400, www.blm.gov/az/ outrec/camping/ camping.htm
OPEN:	Year-round
SITES:	10 plus overflow
EACH SITE:	Picnic table, fire ring
ASSIGNMENT:	First come, first served; no reservations
REGISTRATION:	On-site self-registration
FACILITIES:	Flush toilets, water spigots, drinking fountains
PARKING:	At campsites
FEE:	$5; $5 day use
ELEVATION:	3,500 feet
RESTRICTIONS:	*Pets:* On leash only, pets prohibited in the wilderness *Fires:* In fire rings only; cutting firewood from standing live or dead vegetation prohibited *Alcohol:* Permitted *Vehicles:* 30-foot length limit; 2 vehicles per site *Other:* 14-day stay limit; discharging of firearms prohibited; cleaning game in campground prohibited; checkout 2 p.m., quiet hours 10 p.m.–6 a.m.

MAP

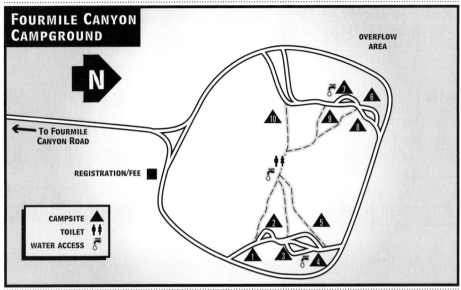

FOURMILE CANYON CAMPGROUND

N

OVERFLOW AREA

TO FOURMILE CANYON ROAD

REGISTRATION/FEE ■

CAMPSITE ▲
TOILET ♀♂
WATER ACCESS ♨

GETTING THERE

From Safford, take US 70 northwest 15 miles to the Aravaipa-Klondyke Road. Turn left and drive southwest 24.5 miles to the junction with the Bonita-Klondyke Road. Turn right and continue northwest 7.5 miles to Klondyke and Fourmile Canyon Road. Turn left and drive southwest 0.5 miles to the campground.

GPS COORDINATES

Zone 12S
Easting 561235
Northing 3632625
North 32° 49' 47.82"
West 110° 20' 44.70"

severely disturbing the primitive camping area near the Turkey Creek trailhead. Plans to fix the road are on hold, but if you can get to the Turkey Creek trail, you can hike to and explore a Salado cliff dwelling without a permit.

With your base at Fourmile, you're in a great position to explore two more of Arizona's most remote wildlands. To the northeast is the Santa Theresa Wilderness, characterized by deep, secretive canyons; high, bare ridgelines; and strikingly sculpted granite outcrops. Human presence here is limited to a few rarely used stock trails and a handful of intrepid backpackers, increasing your chances of observing a peregrine falcon, bighorn sheep, black bear, or mountain lion. The 76,000-acre Galiuro Wilderness stretches off to the southwest, mountainsides green with oak and ponderosa. Hike up Rattlesnake Canyon to Powers Garden, and visit the cabin and mine where the unfortunate Power family shot it out with a posse from Safford in 1918. Trails comb the Galiuros, but the little-used tracks can be faint; bring good maps, a compass, and plenty of water, and check in with the Coronado National Forest Safford Ranger District for more information.

41
RIVERVIEW
CAMPGROUND

THE GILA BOX NATIONAL RIPARIAN CONSERVA-
TION AREA (NRCA) was designated in 1990,
one of only two such areas in the nation. Gila
River and Bonita Creek form a 35-mile corridor of
rare and precious habitat filled with plant and animal
life. Along the water, massive cottonwoods, broad-
leaved sycamores, and willow and walnut trees shade
lush banks, rocky riffles, and sandy beaches. In the
box, sheer cliffs rise above the river, exposed rock layers telling the tale of aeons of intermittent volcanic
upheaval.

Two campgrounds bookend the Gila Box—Owl
Creek on the eastern end and Riverview on the west—
about 23 river-miles downstream. Both are on desert
terrain just outside the fragile riparian corridor, with
views of the Gila winding below. If you're a paddler,
leave your shuttle car at Dry Canyon Boat Take Out
and spend the night at Owl Creek. Head downstream
in the morning to get the best of what the Box has to
offer. If the river's flowing fast, you can make it a day
trip, or dawdle a bit and spend a night along the way.
Primitive camping is allowed throughout the NRCA,
with restrictions in the riparian zone. Visit the U.S.
Geological Survey Web site at **waterdata.usgs.gov/
az/nwis/current/?type=flow** to check current water
flow and contact the Bureau of Land Management for
information and regulations.

If you can't do the full float or you've got other
activities in mind, make your base at the Riverview
Campground. The desert is a little greener here than at
Owl Creek, the sites are farther apart, and river access
is easier. The road in is partially paved, and while it's
quite curvy, it's perfectly passable. This is one of the
newer campgrounds we've seen, and while it may have
less charm than an old CCC site, it's also seen 70 fewer
years of wear and tear. The fire rings are clearly new

*Drift down the Gila
River, maybe with a
fishing line dangling
behind you to tempt
the enormous channel
catfish.*

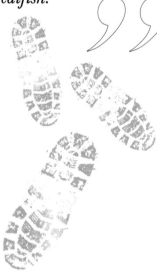

RATINGS

Beauty: ✰ ✰ ✰
Privacy: ✰ ✰ ✰ ✰
Spaciousness: ✰ ✰ ✰ ✰
Quiet: ✰ ✰ ✰ ✰ ✰
Security: ✰ ✰ ✰ ✰
Cleanliness: ✰ ✰ ✰ ✰

KEY INFORMATION

ADDRESS: Safford Field Office
711 14th Avenue
Safford, AZ 85546

OPERATED BY: Bureau of Land Management

INFORMATION: (928) 348-4400, www.blm.gov/az/outrec/camping/camping.htm

OPEN: Year-round

SITES: 13

EACH SITE: Picnic table, fire ring, upright grill, shade ramada

ASSIGNMENT: First come, first served; no reservations

REGISTRATION: On-site self-registration

FACILITIES: Vault toilets; water spigots

PARKING: At campsites

FEE: $5, $3 per person to float, $2 additional vehicle

ELEVATION: 3,300 feet

RESTRICTIONS: *Pets:* On leash only
Fires: In fire rings only
Alcohol: Permitted
Vehicles: No length limit; 2 vehicles per site
Other: 14-day stay limit; quiet hours 10 p.m.–6 a.m.; downed and dead firewood collection only; discharging of firearms prohibited; checkout time 11 a.m.; glass containers prohibited in or along shorelines or creeks

with attached grills that move easily, and the sturdy concrete picnic tables show no abuse. Riverview sites also come complete with upright grills for barbecuing and a small shade ramada to tame the midday sun.

The first seven sites are all very similar, lined up about 200 feet apart and at least that far from the road, overlooking the canyon. Opposite, the sheer cliffs rise 500 feet from the river, reflecting the sound of rushing water. Each site follows the same pattern, with ramada and picnic table in the center, fire ring on the left and grill on the right. Between the sites, prickly pear, ocotillo, mesquite, paloverde, creosote, barrel cactus, and cholla thrive. Due to the rocky ground and the profusion of spiny plants, you'll be most comfortable tenting (with a good mattress under you) in the generous gravel area.

Sites 8 through 13 follow the looping road that mimics the bend in the canyon, and all except 12 and 13 have a view of the river to the west. Site 8 is a wide site on the corner where the road branches off to the river-access and day-use areas, and could easily accommodate a large group. Tall ocotillos surround site 10, the tips of their branches ready to burst into flame with spring blossoms. The last three sites have pull-throughs, and site 11 best suits pop-ups or truck campers since it's the only one without a tent spot of any kind. One set of toilets serves the campground, and it's quite a hike from sites 7, 8, and 9. If you're concerned about making the trek in the middle of the night, consider sites 2, 3, or 13.

At this elevation, desert camping means hot, hot summers and cold winter nights. Come in March for the wildflower bloom, or in fall to hike the canyon bottom under cottonwoods and sycamores blazing with color; in either season you'll find a plethora of migrating birds taking advantage of the oasis. Golden eagles soar year-round, and canyon natives include beaver, javelina, and bighorn sheep. If you're lucky, you may glimpse a mountain lion.

The best hiking is along the watercourses, although high water in the Gila may restrict how far you can safely go. From Riverview, you've got a good base to explore Bonita Creek, where native fish still predominate in the perennial stream. For nonhikers, the Bonita Creek Watchable Wildlife area provides an accessible

MAP

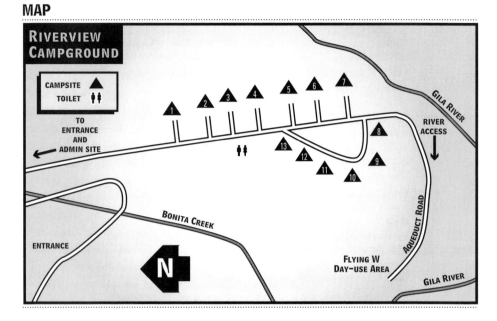

RIVERVIEW CAMPGROUND

CAMPSITE ▲
TOILET 👫

TO ENTRANCE AND ADMIN SITE ←

1 2 3 4 5 6 7 8 9 10 11 12 13

GILA RIVER

RIVER ACCESS

AQUEDUCT ROAD

BONITA CREEK

ENTRANCE

N

FLYING W DAY–USE AREA

GILA RIVER

place to sit and overlook the canyon, and is a great perch to look for birds in the leafy canopy. The Serna Cabin picnic area nearby will help you imagine river-bottom life. Hohokam, Mogollon, Anasazi, and Apache all hunted and farmed in these narrow canyons over the last millennium, and the box was a well-known route for travelers. Early in the 20th century, more than 40 small family farms dotted what is now the NRCA, the Serna homestead among them.

If you've brought your boat but aren't up for an long trip, you can put in at Riverview and drift down to the Dry Canyon Boat Take Out, maybe with a fishing line dangling behind you to tempt the Gila's enormous channel catfish. If land-based recreation is more your thing, you'll find miles and miles of scenic back roads in and around the Gila Box, ranging from well-maintained to quite primitive.

GETTING THERE

From Safford, take US 70 east 5 miles to Sanchez Road. Turn left and head northeast 12 miles, following the signs to the campground.

GPS COORDINATES

Zone 12S
Easting 641968
Northing 3640210
North 32° 53' 27.12"
West 109° 28' 55.92"

42
HOSPITAL FLAT
CAMPGROUND

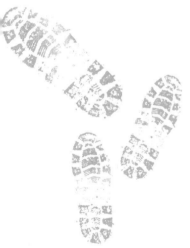

> *Cool temperatures and a beautiful alpine setting are therapeutic.*

DRIVING THE 35 MILES UP THE SWIFT TRAIL from 2,900 feet elevation to 9,000 feet is ecologically comparable to driving from Mexico to Canada. The road winds its way up the Pinaleño Mountains through saguaros and ocotillos to juniper and pinyons and eventually up to the ferns and towering pines. The *Pinaleños* (a mixed Apache/Spanish coinage meaning "many deer") are considered a sky island, with the highest peak, Mount Graham, reaching 10,720 feet. The ecosystem at the top of the mountains is so different than the lower desert that the plants and animals here are almost completely isolated from similar populations in other regions. A tremendous variety of wildlife thrive throughout the mountains, and 18 native species have developed here that cannot be found anywhere else.

The Swift Trail, named after the first supervisor of the Coronado National Forest, turns to dirt after 22 miles and closes at this point during the winter season. There are six campgrounds and two picnic areas along the drive, and several opportunities to get out of the car and enjoy the views over the San Simon and Sulphur Springs valleys. Stop at the Safford Ranger District Office for the route's self-guided tour brochure. The mountain has been a summer retreat since the days of the pioneers, and the Civilian Conservation Corps helped build the roads, campgrounds, and picnic areas. Noon Creek, so named because it was the farthest pioneers were able to get by noon on the first day of a journey up the mountain, is the perfect place to have a picnic and ponder the past.

Just 1 mile beyond the winter gate is Hospital Flat. In the 1880s this meadow was a field hospital for soldiers from Fort Grant, in the western foothills of Mt. Graham. The cool temperatures and beautiful alpine setting were therapeutic for soldiers recovering from hard service in

RATINGS

Beauty: ✩ ✩ ✩ ✩
Privacy: ✩ ✩ ✩ ✩
Spaciousness: ✩ ✩ ✩
Quiet: ✩ ✩ ✩
Security: ✩ ✩ ✩
Cleanliness: ✩ ✩ ✩

the Apache Wars. The hospital also served as a summer haven for officers and their families. The army operated a signal station from nearby Heliograph Peak. Fort Grant remained in service through the Spanish-American War, then was ceded to Arizona upon statehood and became the State Industrial School for Wayward Boys and Girls; it remains a prison today.

Hospital Flat is the only campground along the Swift Trail designated tent-only. All but two sites are set back at least 50 yards from the parking area, requiring a short hike in to your camp. The sites are in the treeline at the edge of a grassy dell filled with bluebells, harebells, and sneezeweed (a lovely little sunflower). A small creek that runs through the meadow must be traversed to get to most of the sites. Sites 10 and 11 combine to form an open and spacious group site, close enough to the parking area that you don't have to worry about hauling your gear or making a midnight hike to the restroom. Sites 8 and 9 are farthest away, downstream where the meadow ends and a small footbridge helps with the sometimes-soggy stream crossing. Site 8 is on the meadow side, with a view and small tent area. A slight rise separates it from site 9, which faces the woods and the starting point of a self-guided nature trail built by the Safford Rotary Club. The 0.75-mile loop returns to the campground behind site 5. In either site you fall asleep to the sound of the water gurgling through a small cascade.

Site 7 is a lovely site farther up the meadow from the parking area. It's underneath the trees but doesn't require a creek crossing. One of several faint paths across the meadow leads through site 7 and across the creek to sites 5 and 6. Site 6 is very overgrown and has no picnic table, but site 5 is well screened and shaded with a good, medium-sized tent spot. Our favorite site was 4, which has its own footpath with a small jump over the creek. It's open to great views of the wildflowers in the meadow and provides two sizable tent areas that are shady in the morning. The three remaining sites are closer to the road and harder to reach, but site 2 has a nice, shady tent spot with no stream crossing.

A surprise awaits at the end of the Swift Trail, where 11-acre Riggs Flat Lake is stocked with trout for

ADDRESS:	Safford Ranger District 711 14th Ave., Suite D Safford, AZ 85546
OPERATED BY:	Coronado National Forest
INFORMATION:	(928) 428-4150, www.fs.fed.us/r3/coronado
OPEN:	April 15–November 14, weather and fire conditions permitting
SITES:	11
EACH SITE:	Picnic table, fire ring, bear-resistant box
ASSIGNMENT:	First come, first served; no reservations
REGISTRATION:	On-site self-registration
FACILITIES:	Vault toilets, fire rings, nature trail
PARKING:	At campsites
FEE:	$10
ELEVATION:	9,000 feet
RESTRICTIONS:	*Pets:* On leash only *Fires:* In fire rings only *Alcohol:* Permitted *Vehicles:* No RVs or trailers; limit 2 vehicles per site *Other:* 10 people per site; 14-day stay limit; bear country food-storage restrictions; no drinking water available

MAP

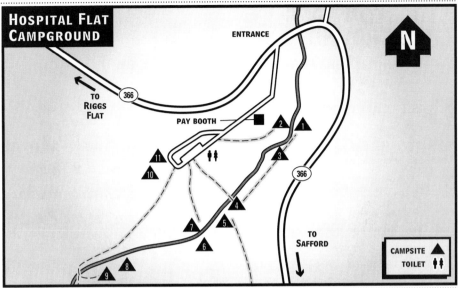

HOSPITAL FLAT CAMPGROUND

ENTRANCE

N

TO RIGGS FLAT

366

PAY BOOTH

2 1

3

366

11

10

4

7 5

6

TO SAFFORD

8

9

CAMPSITE ▲
TOILET ♦♦

GETTING THERE

From Safford, take US 191 south 8 miles to AZ 366. Turn right and drive southwest 23 miles up the mountain and turn left into the campground.

summer fishing. Trails throughout the mountains allow for hiking, biking, and horseback riding, including two relatively new loops specifically developed for mountain bikers.

Atop the highest peak, the Mount Graham International Observatory scans the heavens with some of the world's most sophisticated telescopes. Controversy stirred when the University of Arizona first proposed the observatory, from environmentalists concerned about the habitat of the rare Mount Graham red squirrel, and from Apaches who consider the mountain to have spiritual significance. To find out more and look into the possibility of a tour, stop at Discovery Park on the campus of Eastern Arizona College in Safford.

GPS COORDINATES

Zone 12S
Easting 605643
Northing 3614723
North 32° 39' 54.42"
West 109° 52' 24.18"

43
STOCKTON PASS CAMPGROUND

EASTERN ARIZONA IS THE LAND OF THE THREE C'S: copper, cotton, and cattle, all of which are well represented in the Safford area. Stockton Pass was once the eastern gateway to Aravaipa Canyon and the Sulphur Springs Valley, where the third C reigned supreme. Marshall Trimble, in *Roadside History of Arizona*, called this the "richest cattle country in the West," miles and miles of prime grazing land fed by the rains and snows of the Pinaleño, Galiuro, and Chiricahua mountains. AZ 266 loops around the southern end of the Pinaleños, slipping through Stockton Pass on its way to Bonita, once a thriving town of 1,000 souls. Its ten saloons and several bawdy houses were frequented by prospectors, cowboys, and soldiers from nearby Fort Grant. Today Bonita is a ghost town, Fort Grant is a state prison, and the tall grass that brushed the stirrups of pioneers grows shorter and sparser among prickly pear, sotol, and cholla.

Old Man Stockton, the pass's namesake, ranched in this area in the 1870s. The Forest Service identifies Stockton as father of the Clanton brothers, whose feud with the Earps became American legend when bullets flew at the O.K. Corral. We couldn't find the connection ourselves, but Newman Haynes "Old Man" Clanton, a cattle king (and rumored outlaw boss) who ruled the range from the San Pedro River to the Animas Valley in New Mexico, must certainly have had a stake in this rich area. From the pass, you can look out over the valleys below and imagine the lives of these frontiersmen.

The discreet sign marking the turnoff to the recreation site shows only a picnic table, and casual passersby might not guess that there is a campground tucked back in here. It's this seclusion that appeals to us, as well as the lovely open woodland at the transition between plains and mountain. Eleven sites in seven groups are scattered around the circular parking area,

> *This secluded campground is in a lovely open woodland at the base of the Pinaleño Mountains.*

RATINGS

Beauty: ☆ ☆ ☆
Privacy: ☆ ☆ ☆ ☆
Spaciousness: ☆ ☆ ☆ ☆
Quiet: ☆ ☆ ☆ ☆
Security: ☆ ☆ ☆
Cleanliness: ☆ ☆ ☆

KEY INFORMATION

ADDRESS:	Safford Ranger District 711 14th Ave., Suite D Safford, AZ 85546
OPERATED BY:	Coronado National Forest
INFORMATION:	(928) 428-4150, www.fs.fed.us/r3/coronado
OPEN:	Year-round
SITES:	7
EACH SITE:	Picnic table, fire ring, some have an upright grill
ASSIGNMENT:	First come, first served; no reservations
REGISTRATION:	None required
FACILITIES:	Vault toilets
PARKING:	At campsites, in parking lot
FEE:	Free
ELEVATION:	5,600 feet
RESTRICTIONS:	*Pets:* On leash only *Fires:* In fire rings only *Alcohol:* Permitted *Vehicles:* 16-foot length limit *Other:* 14-day stay limit; bear country food-storage restrictions; no drinking water available

leveled and defined with stonework in characteristic CCC fashion. Mature oak trees and alligator junipers provide shade, and manzanita sprawls between the scattered sites.

The first group of tables (which we take to be site 1/2/3) was once shaded by a mighty oak, although unfortunately all that remains is a mighty stump. This large, sunny area has two fire pits, a large bonfire ring, and plenty of room for lots of tents. It's perfect for families, and even comes with an adorable kid-sized stone picnic table. Going around the loop counter-clockwise, you'll find site 4 convenient to the parking area and the restroom. Set back up a slight rise is 5/6, a double site with two end-to-end picnic tables and two side-by-side fire pits. Nearby trees provide some early-morning or late-afternoon relief, but these are sunny sites at midday.

For deeper shade, choose 7/8, another double site that sits two steps down in a sunken-living-room arrange-ment. Make sure you've got a good ground cloth if there's rain threatening—things could get a little soggy here. A large alligator juniper shades site 9, and in drier weather there's good tenting in the sandy wash next to the site. Follow the path leading under the canopy of trees behind site 9 and you'll find enchanting and secre-tive site 10. There's afternoon shade, a large, bermed tent spot, and an added upright grill. The last site, 11, backs up against a hillside just off its own parking tab, under the shade of a large oak tree. The site itself is compact, level, and nicely laid out, although the tent spots are small and uneven.

Above the grassy slopes to the north loom the pine-capped Pinaleños. The Shake Trail climbs steadily from the campground, up 3,000 feet in less than 5 miles, meeting the Swift Trail near the ridgeline. The effort takes you to beautiful mountain meadows and into deep evergreen forest. Hike up or down with a car shuttle, but you'll need a good guide to help you find the unmarked upper trailhead. Stockton Pass makes a good base to explore the mountains, with far less traffic than the busy campgrounds along the Swift Trail (for more about the Pinaleños, see profile 42, Hospital Flat Campground).

MAP

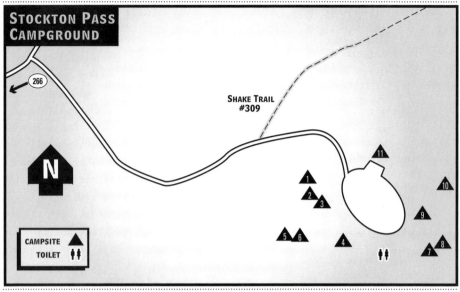

STOCKTON PASS
CAMPGROUND

266

SHAKE TRAIL
#309

N

CAMPSITE
TOILET

The edge is off the summer heat here at 5,600 feet, although you'll still appreciate what shade you can find. Spring is really the season to visit, when the hills are carpeted with wildflowers. Fall can also be very pleasant, even when snow has already brushed the peaks; winter campers should come prepared for cold nights. There are black bears aplenty in the Pinaleños, so keep a clean camp and don't attract a wanderer. Mule deer also pick their delicate way through the campground, and skunks and squirrels abound. It's quiet here, so enjoy nature's night sounds, but don't be alarmed: the weird, plaintive bawling drowning out the coyotes is only lowing cattle. Remember your telescope, too, because once the sun goes down, you'll see why the Pinaleño Mountains host the Mount Graham International Observatory. If you start to feel too lonesome in this remote area, you can backtrack to US 191 and stop at Roper Lake State Park, which offers fine fishing, rental cabins, and a natural hot spring tub.

GETTING THERE

From Safford, take US 191 south 17 miles to AZ 266. Turn right and go west 12 miles to campground entrance. Turn right into the campground.

GPS COORDINATES

Zone 12S

Easting 607452

Northing 3606625

North 32° 35' 30.84"

West 109° 51' 18.06"

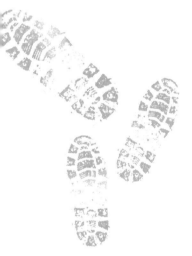

The four camping areas here each have their own persinality.

THE SANTA CATALINA MOUNTAINS are one of Arizona's sky islands—isolated mountains rising thousands of feet above the surrounding sea of desert. They are moist, green havens for plants and animals unable to tolerate the searing heat below and now left stranded by millennia of climate change. Biologists say the 28-mile drive from Tucson to the top of Mount Lemmon is, ecologically, like a trip from Mexico to Canada. Awaking to fog and mist at Spencer Canyon Campground, we certainly felt like we could be in Washington, until we realized we were just inside a cloud.

The Catalina Highway is a designated scenic drive—the Sky Island Parkway—and is a Tucsonian's only access to this cool respite from summer's heat. The route is so popular that the Coronado National Forest requires a day-use fee just to take the drive, unless you're headed specifically for the mountaintop town of Summerhaven or the slopes of Ski Valley. The fees help maintain and improve the facilities, and if you have an interagency access pass, you're covered. As you start to climb, the Tucson valley sprawls out below you and canyons ripple off into the distance like sand shaped by the ocean waves. Pull over and enjoy the view from the Babad Do'ag Vista, which is a great spot to watch the sunset and see the city lights brighten the night.

You can make several neat stops along the drive, including the interpretive trail at Gordon Hirabayashi Campground, once a minimum-security federal "honor camp." The Catalina Highway was built primarily by the men who served their sentences here. If there's been rain lately, the Seven Cataracts Vista lets you peek at the seven waterfalls of Sabino Canyon. A 7.8-mile hike originating in the Sabino Canyon Recreation Area will take you to the base of the cataracts—after 50-plus wet stream crossings.

RATINGS

Beauty: ✩ ✩ ✩
Privacy: ✩ ✩ ✩
Spaciousness: ✩ ✩ ✩
Quiet: ✩ ✩ ✩
Security: ✩ ✩ ✩
Cleanliness: ✩ ✩ ✩ ✩

Farther up, unpack your tackle for Rose Canyon Lake, a seven-acre no-boating lake stocked with rainbow trout, and one of the most popular places on the mountain. The 76 somewhat-crowded campsites here are heavily used and fill up early. At Spencer Canyon Campground, the highest of the area's five campgrounds at 8,000 feet, the host brags that once regulars spend a night here, they won't pitch their tents anywhere else.

Enjoy your trip up the mountain, but don't tarry too long. Many of the campsites at Spencer Canyon are far enough off the road that they'd be difficult to find after dark. There are four camping areas—Ponderosa Loop, East Fork, Spencer Loop, and Turkey Track—and two sets of campground hosts. It's almost as if there are four different campgrounds, each with its own personality. Ponderosa Loop is the first and smallest with seven sites, two of which belong to the resident camp hosts. Sites 6 and 7 are well apart, downhill from the road among the tall pines. At East Fork, nine walk-in sites dot a rocky patch of forest. Site 16 is cute and private, with a fine hearth built into the boulders.

The camp host let slip that, if someone reports rambunctious campers, they expect it to be in Spencer Loop, the largest of the four areas. Despite its bad-boy reputation, Spencer offers several good sites on the slopes among the ponderosas. You may have to hunt for the leveled tent spot in the steeper sites—it's often uphill. Many of the sites throughout Spencer Canyon have steep, tricky access, so keep your flashlight handy.

Turkey Track is farthest in, with several great sites and our favorite spot—site 57. This large, private site is at the end of the loop, hidden past sites 56 and 58. A short hike from here takes you to your own rocky overlook, where you can see the city lights of Tucson miles below.

Between Rose and Spencer canyons, you pass the Forest Service Palisade Visitor Center, the place to find information on all the terrific hikes in the 56,933-acre Pusch Ridge Wilderness, as well as local wildlife. Deer are everywhere, along with fancy Abert's squirrels and nosy Steller's jays; black bears and mountain lions also prowl here.

KEY INFORMATION

ADDRESS: Santa Catalina Ranger District 5700 North Sabino Canyon Rd. Tucson, AZ 85750

OPERATED BY: Coronado National Forest

INFORMATION: (520) 749-8700, www.fs.fed.us/r3/coronado

OPEN: April–October 15

SITES: 66

EACH SITE: Picnic table, fire ring, some have standing grill, bear box

ASSIGNMENT: First come, first served; no reservations

REGISTRATION: On-site self-registration

FACILITIES: Vault toilets, water spigots, campground host, firewood

PARKING: At campsites

FEE: $18 plus $5 recreation area fee, $8 additional vehicle

ELEVATION: 8,000 feet

RESTRICTIONS: *Pets:* On leash only; prohibited in the Pusch Ridge Wilderness *Fires:* In fire rings *Alcohol:* Permitted *Vehicles:* 16-foot length limit; ATVs prohibited, motorized vehicles and bicycles prohibited in Pusch Ridge Wilderness *Other:* 14-day stay limit; bear country food-storage restrictions; firearms prohibited; horses prohibited

MAP

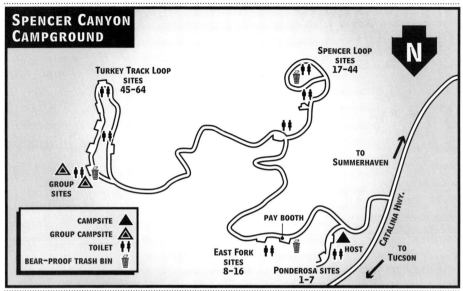

SPENCER CANYON CAMPGROUND

N

SPENCER LOOP SITES 17–44

TURKEY TRACK LOOP SITES 45–64

TO SUMMERHAVEN

GROUP SITES

CAMPSITE ▲
GROUP CAMPSITE △
TOILET ♦♦
BEAR–PROOF TRASH BIN ⬛

PAY BOOTH

EAST FORK SITES 8–16

PONDEROSA SITES 1–7

HOST

TO TUCSON

CATALINA HWY.

GETTING THERE

From Tucson, go east on Tanque Verde to Catalina Highway. Turn left and travel north 4.2 miles to the National Forest boundary. Continue up Mount Lemmon 21 miles to the campground entrance. Turn left into the campground.

GPS COORDINATES

Zone 12S

Easting 524592

Northing 3586859

North 32° 25' 06.72"

West 110° 44' 18.42"

At the top of the mountain lies the town of Summerhaven, which is making an amazing recovery from the devastating Aspen fire of 2003. Stop by the General Store for some homemade fudge and souvenirs, or dine at the Mt. Lemmon Cafe. After a chilly evening in camp, you can also have a warm breakfast at the Iron Door Mine Restaurant in Ski Valley and take a scenic ski-lift ride.

Be prepared for heavy rains during the months of July through September and bring your long johns in spring and fall. It's hard to imagine freezing when it's 80°F in the desert, but on one March trip we saw people shoveling snow into the beds of their pickups to haul it back to Tucson.

For an adventurous trip home, take the Control Road (FR 38) to Oracle down the north side of the mountains. When I asked at the General Store if the Oracle Road was open, the grinning clerk replied, "Sure—if you have a rental car." The road can be steep, narrow, and rough, and four-wheel drive is recommended, but it is a lovely drive.

ALAMO CANYON PRIMITIVE CAMPGROUND

ONE IMAGE, ONE DISTINCTIVE SILHOUETTE, embodies the desert Southwest for people across the globe. From cheesy tourist tchotchkes to the Arizona state quarter, the mighty saguaro raises its arms on high. Arizona has more than one spectacular giant, however, and the extreme southern edge of the state is the one place in the United States where you can admire the massive organ pipe cactus.

Organ Pipe Cactus National Monument preserves and celebrates more than just these prickly behemoths. Plants from five distinctive Sonoran Desert vegetation zones comingle within the park, with upland and lowland species meeting wanderers from the Gulf Coast normally exclusive to Mexico. Many animals have also adapted to this sere and severe environment, including desert bighorn sheep and critically endangered Sonoran pronghorn antelope.

Unfortunately, one of the first questions we hear when Organ Pipe is mentioned is "Is it safe?" The park shares its southern border with Mexico, and El Camino del Diablo, or The Devil's Highway, has been part of an east-to-west route across this almost waterless land since human beings first set foot here. Given its ominous name by Spanish explorers, marked and unmarked graves of travelers from every era dot the trail. Desperados and the simply desperate still travel this road, and increased enforcement in developed areas has pushed more and more traffic in drugs and human labor into remote regions, further imperiling the delicate wilderness the park was established to protect. The park's visitor center is named for Kris Eggle, a ranger who lost his life in 2002 confronting drug runners; stop and read his story on the memorial sign near the entrance.

From 2004 to 2006, the National Park Service constructed a heavy-duty vehicle barrier along 23 miles of the park border. While the barrier isn't a perfect solution, it has almost stopped illicit vehicle traffic through

> *At night an astonishing blanket of stars unrolls above you.*

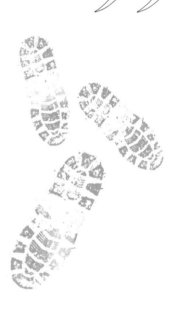

RATINGS

Beauty: ✩ ✩ ✩ ✩
Privacy: ✩ ✩ ✩ ✩
Spaciousness: ✩ ✩ ✩ ✩ ✩
Quiet: ✩ ✩ ✩ ✩ ✩
Security: ✩ ✩ ✩
Cleanliness: ✩ ✩ ✩ ✩

the backcountry, and the long, slow process of recovery has begun for some of the seriously impacted wilderness. There are still backcountry closures in Organ Pipe for visitor safety and resource recovery, but many of the park's nicest hikes and drives are open, and with a modicum of awareness and good sense you'll have a safe and enjoyable visit.

When you first arrive, check in at the visitor center. Your entrance permit is valid for seven consecutive days, and if you have an interagency pass, the fee is waived. Chat with the rangers, pick up information about park activities, browse the books in the gift shop, and check the calendar of ranger patio talks, guided hikes, and van tours.

The 208-site Twin Peaks Campground near the visitor center offers water and flush toilets and is hosted in the winter. At the far end, two rows are designated exclusively for tent campers, with the desert as their backyard, and generators are prohibited in the two rows that separate the larger RVs from the tents. Ocotillo, cholla, and brittlebush abound between sites and stately saguaros and organ pipe cacti stand here and there like sentinels; you'll find several nice spots despite tightly packed arrangement.

Don't settle in yet, though—there's a prime tent-camping opportunity in Organ Pipe for the more self-sufficient. Unless you just like being in the middle of things, head to Alamo Canyon. After making your reservation in person at the visitor center, backtrack north 10 miles on AZ 85 to Alamo Canyon Road. The right turn is not signed, so go slowly and keep your eyes peeled. Drive 3 miles east down the good dirt road to four campsites at the foot of the Ajo Range, whose rugged face glows crimson at sunset due to the rhyolite in the hills.

KEY INFORMATION

ADDRESS:	Organ Pipe Cactus National Monument
	10 Organ Pipe Drive, Ajo, AZ 85321
OPERATED BY:	National Park Service
INFORMATION:	(520) 387-6849, www.nps.gov/orpi
OPEN:	Year-round
SITES:	4
EACH SITE:	Picnic table, upright grill
ASSIGNMENT:	Reservations required and must be made in the visitor center on arrival; reservations can be made only at the visitor center from 9 a.m. to 5 p.m. on the day of the intended stay.
REGISTRATION:	At visitor center
FACILITIES:	Vault toilets, nature trails
PARKING:	At campsites
FEE:	$8 plus $8 entrance fee
ELEVATION:	2,300 feet
RESTRICTIONS:	*Pets:* On leash only, prohibited on some trails; permitted only on Palo Verde and Twin Peaks Campground perimeter trail; prohibited in backcountry. *Fires:* Ground fires and wood fires prohibited. *Alcohol:* Permitted. *Vehicles:* 15-foot length limit; motor homes and trailers prohibited; tent, pickup camper, and vans only; generator use is prohibited. *Other:* 14-day stay limit; discharging of firearms prohibited; firewood gathering prohibited; maximum 20 people per night for the entire campground; quiet hours 10 p.m.–6 a.m.; checkout time is 11 a.m.; bicycles prohibited on foot trails and in backcountry; no drinking water available

MAP

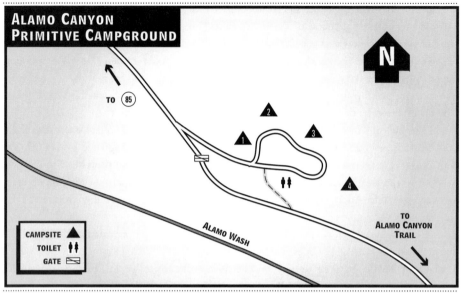

ALAMO CANYON PRIMITIVE CAMPGROUND

TO (85)

N

2

1

3

4

ALAMO WASH

TO
ALAMO CANYON
TRAIL

CAMPSITE ▲
TOILET 👥
GATE ▱

All sites have a picnic table and upright grill, and only site 3 lacks a good tent spot. Saguaros tower around you, and a splendid organ pipe watches over site 2. The pick is spacious site 4, with a great view into Alamo Canyon. At night, an astonishing blanket of stars unrolls above you. And did we mention you have 204 fewer neighbors here?

From this campground you can explore the 1-mile Alamo Canyon Trail. An old ranch house, corrals, and ancient metates testify to centuries of history in the quiet and relatively verdant canyon.

Another way to explore the park is via Ajo Mountain Drive. The 21-mile self-guided loop tour highlights plants indigenous to this area and clues you in to the origins of geologic and geographic features. You can also hike the 4.1-mile round-trip Estes Canyon–Bull Pasture trails for panoramic views and possibly a sighting of bighorn sheep or javelina.

From May to September, daytime temperatures often reach above triple digits, so most visitors come from October through April. Expect Alamo Canyon sites to fill up early in winter months.

GETTING THERE

From Ajo, take AZ 85 south 33 miles through Why to the Kris Eggle Visitor Center.

GPS COORDINATES

Zone 12S

Easting 332533

Northing 3551945

North 32° 5′ 29.04″

West 112° 46′ 28.62″

> *Rare birds can be seen in this riparian oasis.*

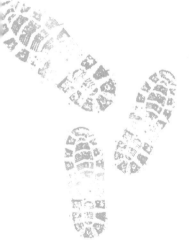

BRING YOUR BINOCULARS AND FIELD GUIDE, because this is the place to go for world-famous bird-watching. At the base of the Santa Rita Mountains, with Mt. Wrightson towering 9,453 feet above, Bog Springs Campground is a bird-watcher's haven set among yucca, oak, and alligator juniper. Riparian Madera Canyon is close enough to Mexico that birds rarely seen north of the border, such as the elegant trogon, visit here during the breeding season. Once heavily logged—*madera* is Spanish for timber— the forest now hosts more than 240 species, including the magnificent hummingbird, the Montezuma quail, and even the rare eared quetzal.

Bog Springs Campground is open year-round, but only hosted during winter months. Come early in the day in April and May, since the campground routinely fills up when migrating birds are in breeding plumage. The 13 sites are arranged in a one-way loop on a hillside, with the flattest and most accessible site, 11, the first one you come to. Site 12, set well below the road in the oaks, provides three good tenting possibilities, while site 13, near the Bog and Kent Springs trailhead, sits on a pair of leveled pads on a steeper slope. Inside of the loop, site 8 has a bit of a view of Green Valley below, but the tent area at site 9 seems to be on the trail to the restrooms. Site 7, at the end of the loop, can accommodate a large RV, but also offers a good tent spot next to the picnic table. Near the restrooms and trailhead parking area, a short flight of steps leads down to three shady sites. Site 6 has a well-built tent pad, and sites 4 and 5 are close enough together to accommodate a larger family. Across the road, sites 2 and 3 combine to make a double, with two picnic tables, two fire pits, and a shared bear box; good for groups or two families camping together. Site 1, compact and rocky, is just across the

RATINGS

Beauty: ✿ ✿ ✿ ✿
Privacy: ✿ ✿ ✿
Spaciousness: ✿ ✿ ✿
Quiet: ✿ ✿ ✿ ✿
Security: ✿ ✿ ✿ ✿
Cleanliness: ✿ ✿ ✿ ✿

Dutch John Spring Trail. The host's trailer is in a separate area, across the camp road from site 4.

Even if bird-watching isn't your thing, the area is rich with other opportunities. Stop at the gatehouse on your way to the campground and pick up a brochure describing local hikes. It's published by the Friends of Madera Canyon, a nonprofit organization that helps the Forest Service maintain the local trails and preserve the canyon. The group has also provided great display maps at the two trailheads in the campground. The Dutch John Spring Trail climbs 1,200 feet in a little less than 2 miles through sycamores and unusually large oaks to two springs. The Bog Springs and Kent Spring trails begin together near site 13 and can be combined to make a nice 4.5-mile loop along a creek. Drive up to the Mt. Wrightson Picnic Area for the difficult 10.8-mile Old Baldy Trail all the way to the peak of Mt. Wrightson; 32 switchbacks on the last stretch will make you work for the 360-degree view. If you don't have an interagency pass, there's a $5 day-use fee per vehicle.

If you want to treat yourself to a night under a roof, the Santa Rita Lodge offers rental cabins, as well as guided bird tours and benches to watch our feathered friends at the bird feeders. Head a little farther south on Interstate 19 to reach the Whipple Observatory via the Mt. Hopkins scenic drive. This partnership between the Smithsonian Institution and University of Arizona offers day-long tours of the 6.5-meter MMT, one of the world's largest optical telescopes. Reservations are required for tours, but you can stop at the visitor center any weekday. If you plan your trip well, you can catch one of their quarterly Saturday star parties, when amateur astronomers set up dozens of telescopes, some homemade, to share the moon, planets, and other galaxies with you. Box Canyon Road scenic drive will take you across the mountains to AZ 83. From here, you can reach the 14.3-mile Santa Rita section of the Arizona Trail, a network of trails beginning at the Mexican border and traversing Arizona lengthwise. The mountains also offer spelunking opportunities in Onyx Cave and the Cave of the Bells. Both caves require permits and advance reservations to enter and are not for beginning cavers.

KEY INFORMATION

ADDRESS: Nogales Ranger District
303 Old Tucson Rd.
Nogales, AZ 85621

OPERATED BY: Coronado National Forest

INFORMATION: (520) 281-2296, www.fs.fed.us/r3/coronado

OPEN: Year-round

SITES: 13

EACH SITE: Picnic table, fire ring, bear-resistant box, some have water spigots, some have bear-proof trash containers

ASSIGNMENT: First come, first served; no reservations

REGISTRATION: On-site self-registration

FACILITIES: Vault toilets, water spigots, campground host

PARKING: At campsites

FEE: $10; $5 day use

ELEVATION: 5,200 feet

RESTRICTIONS: *Pets:* On leash only
Fires: In fire rings only
Alcohol: Permitted
Vehicles: 22-foot length limit; 2 vehicles per site
Other: 14-day stay limit; bear country food-storage restrictions; firearms prohibited; 10 people per site; horses prohibited

MAP

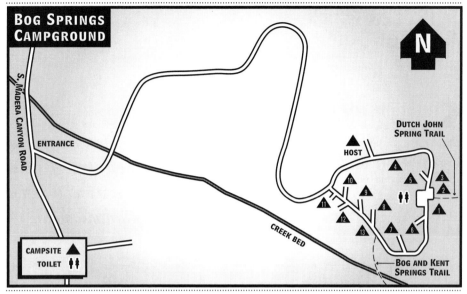

BOG SPRINGS CAMPGROUND

N

S. MADERA CANYON ROAD

ENTRANCE

DUTCH JOHN SPRING TRAIL

HOST

CREEK BED

CAMPSITE ▲
TOILET ♀♂

BOG AND KENT SPRINGS TRAIL

GETTING THERE

From Tucson, take I-19 south 24 miles to Continental Road/Madera Canyon exit (exit 63). Turn left and drive 1 mile to Whitehouse Road. Turn right and continue southeast 11 miles to the campground entrance. Turn left and drive 0.5 miles to the campground.

GPS COORDINATES

Zone 12R
Easting 511310
Northing 3510225
North 31° 43' 38.58"
West 110° 52' 50.22"

Down AZ 83 lies Sonoita. This tiny town, which is not much more than you can see from the four-way stop, is known for its wine. You may be surprised to learn that the soil in this part of Arizona is remarkably similar to the Burgundy region of France, and several successful wineries (which all host tours and tastings) have sprouted up here. This is yet another unique landscape in Arizona; a Hollywood producer thought these rolling, grassy hills looked more like the Midwest than the Midwest itself, and the movie *Oklahoma!* was filmed here. Complete your southern Arizona tour with a stop in Patagonia to cruise the art galleries, stroll through the oldest cottonwoods in the state at Patagonia-Sonoita Creek Preserve, have a slice of pizza at the Velvet Elvis Pizza Company, and take a guided bird-watching boat tour at Patagonia Lake State Park.

47
RUSTLER PARK CAMPGROUND

SET IN THE SOUTHEASTERN CORNER OF THE STATE, the Chiricahua Mountains are one of the most interesting of Arizona's sky islands. On one end hoodoos rise into the sky in weird and unnatural shapes and on the other end laughing streams host exotic bird species in brilliant colors rarely seen north of Mexico. In between, miles of hiking trails wind through pine forests and wildflower-filled meadows that are home to deer, black bears, mountain lions, javelina, and coatimundi.

While in the Chiricahuas, be sure to set aside a day to visit the Chiricahua National Monument. Compacted ash laid down by a volcanic eruption 27 million years ago formed the rocks of this area. Erosion in the intervening aeons has created striking stone spires and wild boulder-balancing acts. To get a small taste, drive the 8-mile Bonita Canyon Drive. If you have more time, take a hike and wander through rock formations with names such as Sea Captain, Duck on a Rock, and Punch and Judy. Loop hikes of varying lengths take you through Echo Canyon, Totem Canyon, or into the Heart of Rocks.

The drive to the campground takes you along Pinery Canyon Scenic Drive (Forest Road 42). As you rise in elevation, you leave the grassy plains behind and climb into junipers and oaks and even higher into the pines. You are rewarded with wonderful views of evergreen mountains fading into the distance. The dirt road is passable by standard passenger cars in dry conditions, although high clearance is still recommended. At Onion Saddle, you'll turn onto FR 42D, which leads to a day-use picnic area and parking lot for the Crest Trail. Beyond the winter gate, the road curves into the campground.

Oddly, it seems like you're coming in to the campground from the wrong end—starting with the higher-

> *Revel in miles of hiking trails through pine forests and wildflower-filled meadows.*

RATINGS

Beauty: ✪ ✪ ✪ ✪
Privacy: ✪ ✪ ✪
Spaciousness: ✪ ✪ ✪
Quiet: ✪ ✪ ✪
Security: ✪ ✪ ✪
Cleanliness: ✪ ✪ ✪ ✪

KEY INFORMATION

ADDRESS:	Douglas Ranger District 1192 West Saddleview Rd. Douglas, AZ 85607
OPERATED BY:	Coronado National Forest
INFORMATION:	(520) 364-3468, www.fs.fed.us/r3/coronado
OPEN:	April–October
SITES:	20
EACH SITE:	Picnic table, fire ring, bear-resistant box
ASSIGNMENT:	First come, first served; no reservations
REGISTRATION:	On-site self-registration
FACILITIES:	Vault toilets
PARKING:	At campsites
FEE:	$10
ELEVATION:	8,500 feet
RESTRICTIONS:	*Pets:* On leash only *Fires:* In fire rings only *Alcohol:* Permitted *Vehicles:* 22-foot length limit; 16-foot length limit on road; 2 vehicles per site *Other:* 14-day stay limit; pack in/pack out; bear country food-storage restrictions; discharging of firearms prohibited; horses prohibited; 10 people per site; no drinking water available

numbered sites. The campground road forms a spiral, curling around a hill flanked with ponderosa pines and Douglas fir and capped by sites 1 through 6. The Forest Service claims 25 campsites here, but we only counted 21, including a day-use site just below the trailhead parking. Site 20 perches above the road across from the trailhead. It's got a large tent pad and might be nice for early-start hikers, but its location outside the gate makes you feel as if you're not really in the campground. Sites 14 through 19 form a semicircle around a small parking lot, with a short uphill walk to the sites required. These sites feel a bit more crowded than the rest of the campground, but are still quite nice. Site 14 is compact, a good choice for a two-person tent, with light screening.

Continue along the spiral and check out the wildflower-filled meadow, the campground's focal point. Site 12 is the group site, with five picnic tables, two fire pits, three bear boxes, and not enough level places to put tents. Sites 7 and 11 have good meadow views, but across the road, sites 9 and 10 sit in splendor in the grasses at the tree line, apart from the rest of the campground.

Follow the road as it curves around and uphill and you'll pass another short connector for the Crest Trail. To your left around the small end loop is site 6, which has a nicely secluded feel and a decent medium-sized tent pad. You may spot an occasional hiker on the trail behind the site. We also liked site 4, which is set well back from the road. A large, mysterious concrete slab in site 3 may have been a cabin foundation or a helipad; feel free to make up your own story. From sites 1 and 2 you get a glimpse of the meadow and other sites below you. None of the sites have designated tent pads but almost all have areas that previous campers have used and improved, bedded with a thick layer of pine needles. Short stone walls built into the hillside by the Civilian Conservation Corps (CCC) in the 1930s bracket each campsite, and some sites still have the original hearths. Bear boxes at each site remind you to keep a clean camp, and plenty of nosy, opportunistic skunks are waiting for you to slip up.

Just beyond the meadow are several CCC cabins that have been converted to a Forest Service administrative site/fire station. There's also overflow parking

MAP

RUSTLER PARK CAMPGROUND

CREST TRAIL

N

6
5
4
1
7
8
11
16
17
2
3
15
18
19
20
14
12
13

FR-42D

ENTRANCE

TRAILHEAD PARKING

CAMPSITE ▲
TOILET ♀♂

TO
FOREST SERVICE
ADMINISTRATIVE SITE

for the Crest Trail. The three sections of this hike form a Y along the high ridgelines of the Chiricahuas. The portion that passes Rustler Park can take you on a short-but-steep 1.5-mile jaunt north to Barfoot Lookout for terrific views toward Cochise Stronghold in the Dragoon Mountains and down into Cave Creek Canyon. An equal hike to the south takes you to Bootlegger Saddle, for more views and access to other trails in the Chiricahua Wilderness. As always, watch the weather and be prepared for the extra effort at high elevation.

In case you were wondering, Rustler Park did indeed get its name from outlaws who hid stolen stock in this remote basin while they altered brands and covered their tracks; Bootlegger Saddle probably commemorates other practitioners of free enterprise.

GETTING THERE

From Willcox, take AZ 186 south 31 miles to AZ 181. Turn left and go 3 miles to FR 42. Turn right and drive 12 miles to the Onion Saddle. Turn right onto FR 42D and continue 3 miles to the campground.

GPS COORDINATES

Zone 12R
Easting 662868
Northing 3531351
North 31° 54' 22.92"
West 109° 16' 39.29"

48
IDLEWILDE CAMPGROUND

> *The creek bed is lined with sycamores.*

THERE'S A DEEP MYSTERY in southern Arizona, and if you cross the state on Interstate 10, you'll see the signs—literally. Vivid yellow billboards asking only, "The Thing. What is it?" adorn the roadside from Tucson to New Mexico, alternating with the barrel's end view of a gunfighter, cordially inviting you to Tombstone.

You'll find plenty of mystery in these parts, but some of the most impressive history doesn't involve six-guns and shoot-outs. Head for the Chiricahua Mountains from the west and you can't miss Texas Canyon, whose boulders give you a taste of the geologic dramas that have taken place here. Look to the south for the distinctive two-headed peak of Dos Cabeza Mountains. Farther east, the Chiricahua Mountains tower in the distance, their tallest peak at 9,797 feet. There, 87,700 acres of wilderness top the rugged volcanic sky island, including a wonderland of weathered crevices, precarious balancing rocks, and eerie hoodoos that form Chiricahua National Monument.

Swing around the mountains to the east side, to the tiny town of Portal, and enter the wilderness through Cave Creek Canyon. Make a quick stop at the visitor center to pick up trail information, and make sure to get a bird list. More than 300 bird species make their home in the Chiricahuas, and Cave Creek is famous for its bird-watching.

The first campground you come to is Idlewilde, across a concrete bridge over the perennial creek. Sheer, peach-colored cliffs covered in lime-green lichen shade this canyon campground. The sun won't hit your tent until late morning and the cliffs' height will shorten your evening. The whole campground is lovely, starting with the very first site, set right next to the creek in the shadow of an immense boulder. More granite behemoths shelter and screen many of the sites.

RATINGS

Beauty: ✪ ✪ ✪ ✪
Privacy: ✪ ✪ ✪ ✪
Spaciousness: ✪ ✪ ✪
Quiet: ✪ ✪ ✪
Security: ✪ ✪ ✪
Cleanliness: ✪ ✪ ✪ ✪

Open to the smooth dirt road, sites 3 and 4 are neighborly, good for a large group or a couple of families traveling together. Site 6 requires hiking up a few steps, but you have a nice view of the canyon and a lot of privacy. Sites 7 and 8 also have steps, and the picnic table at site 8 is hidden behind a large boulder. While sites 9 and 10 are near each other, a large granite outcrop separates them; spacious site 10 may be the nicest of them all.

It's just a short walk to the creek from any of the sites, and you can hear the water cascading over the rocks throughout the campground. The creek bed is lined with sycamores with huge leaves and beautifully marbled bark. Arizona cypress, alligator juniper, Arizona madrone, oaks, and the occasional yucca also surround you. In the evening, take a stroll and watch the road for hunting nightjars. Altogether, Idlewilde lives up to its romantic-sounding name.

Just downstream from the campground, the difficult Silver Peak Trail climbs 3,000 feet in just 4.6 miles, to a 7,975-foot summit with breathtaking panoramic views. Less than a mile up the road is the much easier 200-yard Vista Point Trail, a short climb that takes you up and out of the woods for a nice view of the canyon and surrounding mountains. You'll note signs near the trailheads stating that all of the trails in the Douglas Ranger District are in poor condition due to lack of funding, and recommending a letter to your congressman. (Budget cuts are also cited as the reason for seasonal closures at Idlewilde.) Enjoy your hike but keep an eye out for potholes and standing dead timber.

Another sign you'll see throughout southern Arizona reads "Smuggling and illegal immigration may be encountered in this area." While problems are rare for campers and hikers, authorities recommend not hiking alone and avoiding areas where there are well-used unofficial trails and signs of debris from border-crossers.

Cave Creek also boasts South Fork Zoological and Botanical Area, world famous for its bird-watching and wildlife viewing, and well worth the $5 day-use fee. Listen for the barking call of the elegant trogon. This beautiful bird with a bright red belly, white chest band, and brilliant emerald head only enters the United States

KEY INFORMATION

ADDRESS:	Douglas Ranger District 3081 North Leslie Canyon Rd. Douglas, AZ 85607
OPERATED BY:	Coronado National Forest
INFORMATION:	(520) 364-3468, www.fs.fed.us/r3/coronado
OPEN:	May–October
SITES:	10
EACH SITE:	Picnic table, fire ring
ASSIGNMENT:	First come, first served; no reservations
REGISTRATION:	On-site self-registration
FACILITIES:	Vault toilets, water spigots
PARKING:	At campsites
FEE:	$10
ELEVATION:	5,000 feet
RESTRICTIONS:	*Pets:* On leash only *Fires:* In fire rings only *Alcohol:* Permitted *Vehicles:* 16-foot length limit; 2 vehicles per site; motorized/mechanized vehicles not permitted in the Chiricahua Wilderness. *Other:* 14-day stay limit; bear country food-storage restrictions; firearms prohibited; horses prohibited; 10 people per site

MAP

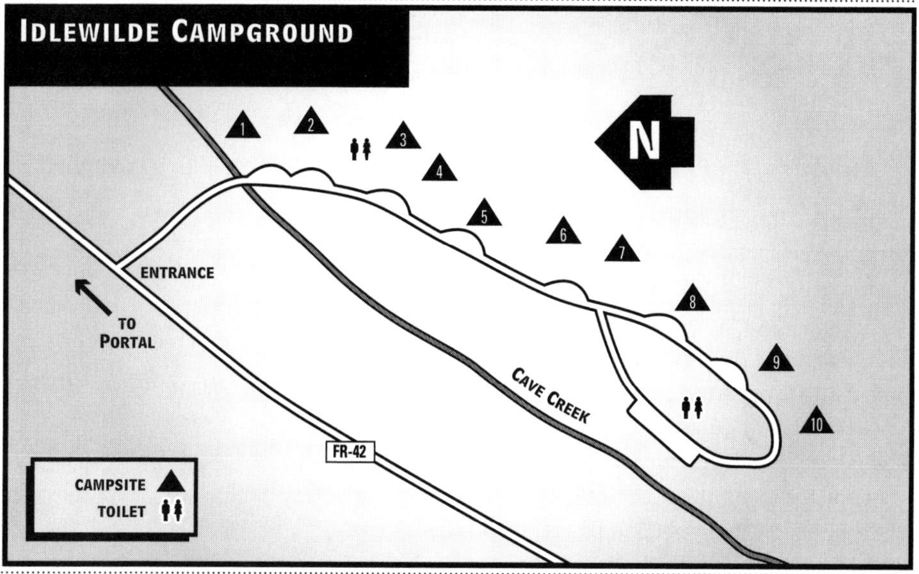

IDLEWILDE CAMPGROUND
N
ENTRANCE
TO PORTAL
CAVE CREEK
FR-42
CAMPSITE
TOILET
1
2
3
4
5
6
7
8
9
10

GETTING THERE

From Tucson, take I-10 east 120 miles to San Simon and Paradise Road (exit 382). Follow the signs for Portal and drive south 22 miles to Paradise. Turn left at FR 42B and drive 5 miles to Portal. Turn right at FR 42 (Cave Creek Road) and continue south 1.5 miles to the campground entrance. Turn left into the campground.

GPS COORDINATES

Zone 12R
Easting 673420
Northing 3530212
North 31° 53' 40.32"
West 109° 9' 58.44"

along the Mexican border, and this is one of the best places to see it. (Professional bird-watchers take note: use of recorded calls to attract the birds is not allowed here during the breeding months.) The American Museum of Natural History's Southwest Research Station is also located nearby. Scientists work here but visitors are welcome to bird-watch—five-day birding tours are available, and volunteers are always needed.

With five campgrounds along Cave Creek Canyon, you shouldn't have a hard time finding a spot even during busy bird-watching months. A vehicle with moderate clearance can drive across the Chiricahuas in good weather, and it's a beautiful back-road trip over to the National Monument. For more details, check out profile 47, Rustler Park Campground.

Are you still wondering about the "Thing"? Well, if you have a taste for the odd, offbeat, kitschy, and slightly hokey, it's well worth the $1 price of admission.

49

LAKEVIEW CAMPGROUND

JUST 7 MILES NORTH of the Mexican border, at the base of the Canelo Hills, sits Parker Canyon Lake. Created by damming the runoff from the Huachuca Mountains, the 132-acre lake now provides bird-watching, boating, and fishing opportunities to anyone wishing to get away from the crowds. The Lakeview Campground, which lives up to its name, has two sections—one for tents and one for RVs. The area specifically for tent campers is on the left as you come in, closer to the shore on a grassy hillside. There you'll find 40 sites spread along two loops, each with a picnic table and a fire pit with grill (some have an upright grill). Head into the right-hand loop but bypass the first ten sites since you can't see the lake as well from there. Sites 14, 18, 19, and 20 are set down the slope toward the water's edge at the end of the loop. If the grass is tall, you may have trouble spotting the tables that are farther away from the road (it took us several minutes to find site 29).

On the other, smaller loop, four sites are arranged above the parking area and six sites a few steps below. You can easily reach the water from any of the sites by hiking down the hillside. This loop has the feel of a converted picnic area. The tables are a little too close together and the sites lack clearly defined tent pads, but even so our favorite site is here—number 32. Spacious, with room for a large tent, it is the farthest down and has a 180-degree view of the lake below. The landscape here is typical of the Upper Sonoran life zone, and the grasslands are dotted with mature junipers and oaks that provide some shade. The summer houses and cabins on the far side of the lake seem strange, since so many of Arizona's lakes are entirely on federal land, but it helps you imagine you've been invited to a private ranch.

If you're more interested in privacy than a view, and if the campground's not very full, take a look at the

> *This site has a 180-degree view of the lake below.*

RATINGS

Beauty: ✩ ✩ ✩ ✩
Privacy: ✩ ✩ ✩
Spaciousness: ✩ ✩ ✩
Quiet: ✩ ✩ ✩
Security: ✩ ✩ ✩
Cleanliness: ✩ ✩ ✩

KEY INFORMATION

ADDRESS: Sierra Vista
Ranger District
5990 South Hwy. 92
Hereford, AZ
85615

OPERATED BY: Coronado
National Forest

INFORMATION: (520) 378-0311,
www.fs.fed.us/r3/
coronado

OPEN: Year-round

SITES: 65

EACH SITE: Picnic table, fire
ring

ASSIGNMENT: First come, first
served; reserva-
tions accepted for
group sites

REGISTRATION: On-site self-
registration

FACILITIES: Vault toilets,
water spigots,
boat ramp, fishing
dock, group sites,
camp host, gen-
eral store, boat
rentals, handicap-
accessible sites

PARKING: At campsites

FEE: $10

ELEVATION: 5,400 feet

RESTRICTIONS: *Pets:* On leash only
Fires: In fire rings
Alcohol: Permitted
Vehicles: No RVs or
trailers in tent
loop; 32-foot limit;
2 vehicles per site;
motorbikes
restricted to
entering/exiting
campsite
Other: 14-day stay
limit; 8-horse-
power boat-motor
limit; bear coun-
try food-storage
restrictions; no
horses

sites across the road. This is nominally the RV section, but some of the sites have nice tent pads and there's a bit more brush for screening and shade. Camping outside of the designated sites is prohibited at Parker Canyon Lake.

Just down the road is the boat ramp and fishing dock. The general store offers a chance to purchase forgotten items, but it is closed on Wednesdays during the summer and from Tuesday through Thursday in the winter. Several boats are available for rent. Parker Canyon Lake makes a good year-round destination, and during hunting season, expect to see the sites filled with camouflaged men. The lake is always popular with fisher folk; rainbow trout, bass, catfish, and sunfish all wait to be lured out of the depths.

The 5-mile Lakeshore Trail #128 travels completely around the lake past cottonwoods, manzanita, and rolling grassy hills. The hike is primarily on level ground, close to the shoreline. Be sure to bring your binoculars and field guide, since you are bound to see a variety of waterfowl and possibly an osprey or an eagle.

The north trailhead of the Arizona Trail's Passage 1 begins at Parker Canyon Lake. From here you can hike 22 miles through the Miller Peak Wilderness to Montezuma Pass, the point along Forest Road 61 where you can reach the other side of the Huachuca Mountains. Passage 2 of the Arizona Trail heads north into the Canelo Hills, connecting with Passage 3 and ending up in Patagonia. Illegal immigration is common in this area, and it is recommended that hikers be aware of their surroundings. Do not camp close to the trail and do not hike alone. Forestry officials also suggest you avoid hiking in the summer since water is scarce and temperatures can be dangerously high. Be prepared for lake-clearing thunderstorms during the summer monsoon months of July through September.

The scenic drive along FR 61 brings you along the southern edge of the Huachuca Mountains with grassy valleys and side canyons below you. From Montezuma Pass, you have a grand overlook of the San Pedro River and San Rafael valleys and—somewhere down there—the international border. You can see more of Mexico than Arizona from here. In 18 miles, the

MAP

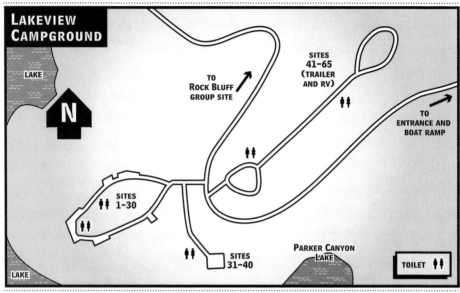

From Sierra Vista, take AZ 92 south 14 miles to the Coronado Memorial Road (FR 61). Turn right and head south and west 16 miles to AZ 83. Veer right and go northwest 5.5 miles to Parker Canyon Lake.

From Tucson, take I-10 to AZ 83. Turn right and continue south through Sonoita 63 miles to Parker Canyon Lake.

drive takes you all the way to the Coronado National Memorial, which commemorates 16th-century Spanish explorer Francisco Vasquez de Coronado's expedition from Mexico into the United States. While hiking through the Coronado National Memorial, it's easy to imagine what it must have been like for Coronado to travel this rugged countryside.

On your way to or from Parker Canyon Lake, be sure to stop at the wineries in Sonoita and Elgin. Here you can taste samples of wine made with grapes grown right here in southern Arizona, and if you happen to be there during the Harvest Festival, you can try stomping on the grapes yourself.

GPS COORDINATES

Zone 12R

Easting 552160

Northing 3477220

North 31° 25' 42.54"

West 110° 27' 04.20"

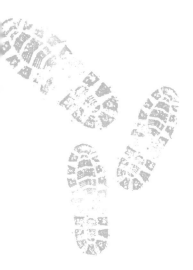

> *Some sites are exactly where miners' cabins once stood.*

FROM SIERRA VISTA, YOU CAN SEE the Huachuca Mountains rising like ramparts behind the fort that shares their name. Enter the mountains on Carr Canyon Road, and shortly you find the Carr House Information Center. This former ranch at the base of the hills, which is open on weekends, offers exhibits on area flora, fauna, and history. You can hike the nature trail at any time. After the information center the road continues, switchbacking up more than 2,000 feet past occasional waterfalls and splendid views over the San Pedro River valley. On your way up, look for the Carr Reef, a band of sheer, white quartzite running along the mountainside. Prospectors looked at this formation and saw dollar signs, since quartzite is often an indicator of gold beneath; in fact, miners harvested gold, silver, tungsten, and quartz from these mountains. The reef gave its name to the mining town that sprang up here, which in turn passed it on to the campground.

Ponderosa pine, alligator juniper, and Douglas fir shade Reef Townsite, while manzanita and silverleaf oak provide screening between the well-spaced sites; according to the Forest Service, some sites are exactly where miners' cabins once stood. The campground is a pair of loops, numbered counterclockwise, with sites 16, 15, 1, and 2 at the higher end of the sloping townsite. Sites 3, 5, 7, 8, and 9 back up to a small wash, which offers a pleasant soundtrack when water is flowing. Surrounded by manzanita, site 14 sits by itself, overlooking sites 12 and 13. The last small loop, and especially site 11, is quite close to the reservable group site. Our favorite is site 10, from which you can climb a short trail to a picnic table at your very own private overlook. Whichever site you choose, a cleared and leveled tent pad makes for a comfortable night.

RATINGS

Beauty: ✿ ✿ ✿ ✿
Privacy: ✿ ✿ ✿
Spaciousness: ✿ ✿ ✿ ✿
Quiet: ✿ ✿ ✿
Security: ✿ ✿ ✿
Cleanliness: ✿ ✿ ✿ ✿

To learn more about the history of Reef, hike the 0.7-mile Reef Historic Trail, which begins and ends near site 10. As interpretive signs describe geologic features and the activities of the Exposed Reef Mining Company, spectacular views of Carr Canyon unfold below. The trail was originally a mining road, and you can compare the landscape you see now with photographs of Reef's mining heyday.

If Reef Townsite Campground is full, or simply not high enough for you, continue to Ramsey Vista Campground. Most of the sites are closer together and more exposed to one another than at Reef Townsite, but sites 1, 2, and 4 on the outside of the loop have particularly good views of Sierra Vista and the San Pedro Valley below. A corral is located near site 1, but horses are not recommended on many of the trails, including Carr Peak Trail. Horses are not permitted in Reef Townsite.

Two trailheads (one across the road from the Reef Townsite Campground entrance, the other just before you get to Ramsey Vista Campground) give you access to the network of trails leading through the Miller Peak Wilderness and up to Carr Peak (9,230 feet) or Miller Peak (9,466 feet). Trails include the Comfort Springs Trail #109, which leaves Ramsey Vista and heads downhill through Carr Canyon and Ramsey Canyon and, if connected with Hamburg Trail #122, all the way to Ramsey Canyon Preserve. Make arrangements to leave a vehicle at the preserve and you can hike all the way down, spend the day at this lush riparian oasis, and drive back up to your campsite.

Because of the canyon's direction, its walls' height, and the occurrence of a spring-fed stream, Ramsey Canyon is wet and cool, making a perfect habitat for a wide variety of plant and animal life. More than 170 bird species are found in the preserve, and the hummingbird observation area is one of the best places to see 17 different species of hummers. Stop by in the morning and catch a guided nature walk; you may catch a glimpse of a coatimundi, a relative of the raccoon found only in the Southwest. The Nature Conservancy manages the preserve and collects a $5 fee per person except on the first Saturday of each month; it's

KEY INFORMATION

ADDRESS: Sierra Vista Ranger District 5990 S. Hwy. 92 Hereford, AZ 85615

OPERATED BY: Coronado National Forest

INFORMATION: (520) 378-0311, www.fs.fed.us/r3/coronado

OPEN: April–November

SITES: 16

EACH SITE: Picnic table, fire ring, some have upright grills

ASSIGNMENT: First come, first served; group site reservations accepted

REGISTRATION: On-site self-registration

FACILITIES: Vault toilets, water spigots

PARKING: At campsites

FEE: $10; $10 day-use, $45 group site

ELEVATION: 7,200 feet

RESTRICTIONS: *Pets:* On leash only
Fires: In fire rings
Alcohol: Permitted
Vehicles: 12-foot trailer limit; 20-foot vehicle limit; 2 vehicles per site; motorized and mechanized vehicles, including mountain bikes, prohibited in wilderness.
Other: 14-day stay limit; bear country food-storage restrictions; firearms prohibited; horses prohibited; 10 people per site; quiet hours 10 p.m.–6 a.m.

MAP

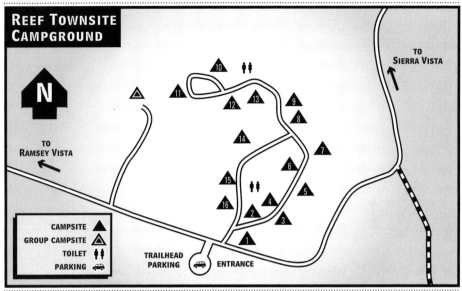

GETTING THERE

From Sierra Vista, take AZ 92 south to Carr Canyon Road. Turn right and continue up the mountain 6.5 miles to the campground entrance.

closed on holidays and on Tuesdays and Wednesdays during the winter.

Save some time in your itinerary to visit Fort Huachuca, which has an unbroken history of military service from 1877 to today. The Fort Huachuca Museum includes exhibits about the Buffalo Soldiers, the campaign against Geronimo, and daily life in the frontier army, while the U.S. Army Intelligence Museum covers more modern aspects of the military mission.

Nearby, San Pedro Riparian National Conservation Area—57,000 acres of land along the San Pedro River—is home to 350 species of birds and more than 80 species of mammals. Check the hike schedule to join guided treks to see Arizona's largest cottonwood, the Hohokam petroglyphs, or the ruins of abandoned mills.

Historic Tombstone, the infamous "Town Too Tough to Die," is also just up the way. There you can relive the gunfight at the O.K. Corral, join a ghost tour of the historic buildings (including the notorious Bird Cage Theatre, now a museum), or have a drink at one of the many saloons.

GPS COORDINATES

Zone 12R

Easting 567403

Northing 3477263

North 31° 25' 41.10"

West 110° 17' 26.82"

APPENDIX A: SOURCES OF INFORMATION

Arizona Game and Fish Department
5000 West Carefree Highway
Phoenix, AZ 85086-5000
(602) 942-3000
www.azgfd.gov

Arizona State Land Department
1616 West Adams Street
Phoenix, AZ 85007
(602) 542-4631
www.land.state.az.us

Arizona State Parks
1300 West Washington
Phoenix, AZ 85007
(602) 542-4174
www.azstateparks.com

Apache-Sitgreaves National Forest
P.O. Box 640
Springerville, AZ 85938
(928) 333-4301
www.fs.fed.us/r3/asnf

Bureau of Land Management
Arizona State Office
One North Central Avenue
Suite 800
Phoenix, AZ 85004-4427
(602) 417-9200
www.az.blm.gov

Coconino National Forest
1824 South Thompson Street
Flagstaff, AZ 86001
(928) 527-3600
www.fs.fed.us/r3/coconino

Coronado National Forest
300 West Congress Street
Tucson, AZ, 85701
(520) 388-8300
www.fs.fed.us/r3/coronado

Grand Canyon National Park
P.O. Box 129
Grand Canyon, AZ 86023
(928) 638-7888
www.nps.gov/grca

Kaibab National Forest
800 South Sixth Street
Williams, AZ 86046
(928) 635-8200
www.fs.fed.us/r3/kai

Maricopa County Parks and Recreation
Department
Headquarters Administrative Offices
234 North Central Avenue, Suite 6400
Phoenix, AZ 85004
(602) 506-2930
www.maricopa.gov/parks

APPENDIX A: SOURCES OF INFORMATION

[continued]

The Nature Conservancy
Phoenix Conservation Center
The Plaza at Squaw Peak III
7600 North 15th Street, #100
Phoenix, AZ 85020
(602) 712-0048
www.nature.org/arizona

Navajo National Monument
HC 71 Box 3
Tonalea, AZ 86044
(928) 672-2700
www.nps.gov/nava

Organ Pipe Cactus National Monument
10 Organ Pipe Drive
Ajo, AZ 85321
(520) 387-6849
www.nps.gov/orpi

Prescott National Forest
344 South Cortez Street
Prescott, AZ 86303
(928) 443-8000
www.fs.fed.us/r3/prescott

Tonto National Forest
2324 East McDowell Road
Phoenix, AZ 85006
(602) 225-5200
www.fs.fed.us/r3/tonto

White Mountain Apache Tribe
Wildlife and Outdoor Recreation Division
100 West Fatco Road
P.O. Box 220
Whiteriver, AZ 85941
(928) 338-4385
www.wmatoutdoors.org

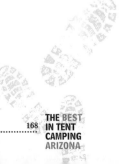

APPENDIX B
CAMPING-EQUIPMENT CHECKLIST

Except for the large and bulky items on this list, I keep a plastic storage container full of the essentials for car camping so they're ready to go when I am. I make a last-minute check of the inventory, resupply anything that's low or missing, and away I go.

COOKING UTENSILS

Aluminum foil
Bottle opener
Can opener
Corkscrew
Cups, plastic or tin
Dish soap (biodegradable), sponge, and towel
Flatware
Frying pan
Fuel for stove
Matches in waterproof container
Plates
Pocketknife
Pot with lid
Salt, pepper, spices, sugar, cooking oil, and maple syrup in spillproof containers
Spatula
Stove
Wooden spoon

FIRST-AID KIT

Antibiotic cream
Band-Aids®
Diphenhydramine (Benadryl®)
Gauze pads
Ibuprofen or aspirin
Insect repellent
Lip balm
Moleskin®
Snakebite kit
Sunscreen
Tape, waterproof adhesive

SLEEPING GEAR

Pillow
Sleeping bag
Sleeping pad, inflatable or insulated
Tent with ground tarp and rainfly

MISCELLANEOUS

Bath soap (biodegradable), washcloth, and towel
Camp chair
Candles
Cooler
Deck of cards
Duct tape
Fire starter
Flashlight or headlamp with fresh batteries
Foul-weather clothing
Paper towels
Plastic zip-top bags
Sunglasses
Toilet paper
Water bottle
Wool or fleece blanket
Optional:
Barbecue grill
Binoculars
Field guides
Fishing rod and tackle
Hatchet
Kayak and related paddling gear
Lantern
Maps (road, topographic, trails, and so on)
Mountain bike and related riding gear

INDEX

GPS OUTDOORS

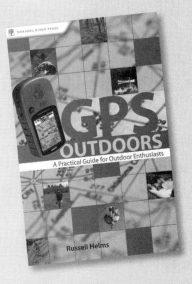

by Russell Helms
ISBN 13: 978-0-89732-967-5
6x9, paperback, $10.95
120 pages: maps, photographs, index

Whether your're a hiker on a weekend trip through the Great Smokies, a back-packer cruising the Continental Divide Trail, a mountain biker kicking up dust in Moab, a paddler running the Lewis and Clark bicentennial route, or a climber pre-scouting the routes up Mount Shasta, a simple handheld GPS unit is fun, useful, and can even be a lifesaver.

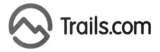
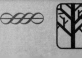 **MENASHA RIDGE PRESS**
www.menasharidge.com

DEAR CUSTOMERS AND FRIENDS,

SUPPORTING YOUR INTEREST IN OUTDOOR ADVENTURE, travel, and an active lifestyle is central to our operations, from the authors we choose to the locations we detail to the way we design our books. Menasha Ridge Press was incorporated in 1982 by a group of veteran outdoorsmen and professional outfitters. For 25 years now, we've specialized in creating books that benefit the outdoors enthusiast.

Almost immediately, Menasha Ridge Press earned a reputation for revolutionizing outdoors- and travel-guidebook publishing. For such activities as canoeing, kayaking, hiking, backpacking, and mountain biking, we established new standards of quality that transformed the whole genre, resulting in outdoor-recreation guides of great sophistication and solid content. Menasha Ridge continues to be outdoor publishing's greatest innovator.

The folks at Menasha Ridge Press are as at home on a white-water river or mountain trail as they are editing a manuscript. The books we build for you are the best they can be, because we're responding to your needs. Plus, we use and depend on them ourselves.

We look forward to seeing you on the river or the trail. If you'd like to contact us directly, join in at www.trekalong.com or visit us at www.menasharidge.com. We thank you for your interest in our books and the natural world around us all.

SAFE TRAVELS,

Bob Sehlinger

BOB SEHLINGER
PUBLISHER